BL

BEDROOM LOGIC

BY

OBI ORAKWUE

BEDROOM POLITICS SERIES

BEDROOM LOGIC

BY

OBI ORAKWUE

Be-Your-Dream-Press

OBRAKE

BEDROOM LOGIC

BY

OBI ORAKWUE

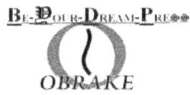

Be Your Dream Press

Imprint of Obrake USA LLC
New York, United States of America

BEDROOM LOGIC

Book Designed by Obrake Designs
Library of Congress Cataloging in Publication Data
Orakwue, Obi
Bedroom Logic/Obi Orakwue
Library of Congress Control Number 2012908995
Includes glossary of terms
ISBN 978-1-948735-03-2 Paperback Edition
ISBN 978-0-9856222-2-0 E-Book Edition
Printed in USA
First Published in USA in 2012, in E-Book Edition
By Be Your Dream Press
Imprint of Obrake USA LLC
New York, United States of America
www.obrake.com

Dedication

This book is dedicated to natural remedies to imperfection, aging and time, and to all the people who aspire to be armed with knowledge to improve their sex drive, enhance their libido and intensify their orgasm, perfecting their sexual pleasure and optimizing their sex life.

Acknowledgments

Thanks to all the people who were involved through research and or interview during the course of writing this book.

TABLE OF CONTENTS

Sexual Desire Disorder

Sexual Dysfunction or Sexual Malfunction

Sexual Desire Disorder

- ✓ Aging
- ✓ Fatigue
- ✓ Pregnancy
- ✓ Medication

Sexual Arousal Disorders

ERECTILE DYSFUNCTION

Causes of Erectile Dysfunction

Damaged or Malfunction of the Nervi Erigentes

Diabetes

FRIGIDITY

Orgasm Disorders or Anorgasmia

Types of Anorgasmia

Primary Anorgasmia

Secondary Anorgasmia

Situational Anorgasmia

Random Anorgasmia

Treatment

Erectile Dysfunction

Female Sexual Dysfunctions

Sexual Pain Disorders

Hypoactive Sexual Desire Disorder (HSDD) or Sexual Aversion Disorder

Medication and Sex Drive

Spinach and Green Vegetables

Pumpkin Seeds

Spicy Chili Peppers

Garlic

Soy And Soy Products

Black Beans and Other Legumes

Basil

Asparagus

Eggs

Brown Rice

Yam

Okra

Crab And Lobsters

Prunes, Hazelnuts, Peanuts, Kiwi, Plum, Pear

Oxytocin

Probable Inducers of Oxytocin

Massage

Exercise

Omega-3 fatty acids

Okra

Chili Pepper

Lettuce

Kelp/Algae/Seaweed

Caviar

Pine Nuts

Mustard Seed

FRUITS

Watermelon

Nutmeg

Pineapple

Blueberries, Raspberries, and Strawberries

Goji Berry

Figs

Dates

Chapter 8

Herbs and Roots to Improve Libido

Manjakani or Oak Gall

Curcuma Comosa

Blackcohosh

Ginseng

Damiana or Wild Yam (extract)

Dong Quai

Epinedium Sagittatum – Horny Goat Weed

Tribulus Terrestries

Hypothetical Side Effect of Tribulus

Other Foods with Estrogen and Estrogen-Like Phytochemicals

Liqourice

Maca Root

Hesperidin

Muira Puama

Saw Palmetto

Whitethorn

Macuna Pruriens

Ashwaganda

Rhodiola Rosea

Kava

Ginkgo Biloba

Catuaba Bark Extract

Chapter 9

Vitamins-Supplements-Minerals For Sex Drive and Libido

Vitamin E

Topical Application of Vitamin E Oil

Vitamin A

Beta-carotene

Elastin

Collagen

Vitamin C

Vitamin D

Vitamin B6

Vitamin B12 + Vitamin B9

Vitamin K

Arginine or L-Arginine

L-Lysine

DHEA

Minerals for Sex Drive and Libido

Magnesium

Selenium

BEDROOM LOGIC

Author's Note

Bedroom politics is complex and the most essential politics of any relationship. However, as complex and intricate as it may be, it has one magic key. The only logical point in the bedroom is healthy and vibrant sex drive, sexual desire, sexual arousal and libido. Once you have healthy libido and sex drive in the bedroom, you have logic. Sex is very essential to any relationship, it is important to sustain a relationship. Once the sex life of a couple is healthy and enjoyable, other existential problems of a relationship may become more easily managed. However, to have a healthy sexual relationship, you need to have the 'Logic' – Sex Drive.

Healthy sex drive and libido may be just a grocery store away. Most active ingredients in the pills for sex drive, sexual desire, sexual arousal and libido are derived from the food, vegetables and plants you see every day. However, you need to know them and know how to eat and employ them to your benefit.

All the points, methods, techniques, foods, vitamins and minerals outlined in this book are not quick fix. Maintaining a healthy and mindful lifestyle and incorporating the foods, herbs and exercise discussed in this edition of the book, in your daily way of life should be a primary focus. The understanding that it is a continuous course of duty and lifestyle will make the intake of these food, herbs, vitamins and minerals to be effective in increasing and maintaining your sexual health. For best result, articulate daily feeding with doing supplements and vitamins. Some of the herbs are better used on intermittent rather than on a daily basis. Again, as said earlier, the methods and techniques are not any quick fix. However, some foods, herbs, vitamins and juices are better taken hours and minutes before any bedroom session.

They take days, weeks, months and years to show a lasting effect. Good thing about the manifestation of the result/effect of the exercise and dietary regimen is that once they manifest, most people can hold on for as long as life permits. Why? Because the more you practice it, the more you will get used to maintaining the healthy dietary lifestyle and regimen.

INTRODUCTION

For practical purposes, the definition of bedroom logic points to one thing: Sex Drive, Sexual Desire, Sexual Arousal and Libido. It is just true that without sex drive and libido, all logic of the bedroom is lost. Healthy sex drive and libido is what some people take for granted especially in our younger years. However, as people grow old, mainly from late twenties, sex drive and libido starts to decrease. The decrease in sex drive, sexual desire, sexual arousal and libido declines with age because age enlists hormonal changes in both men and women. Other factors such as stress, lack of exercise, poor nutrition, and insufficient vitamins and minerals may also be culpable for a person's low sex drive. However, most causes of Low sex drive and libido is curable through dietary regimen, exercise, vitamins, minerals, supplements and hormonal replacement therapy and healthy lifestyle. In this book – Bedroom Logic, you will find most of the steps and techniques to improve and restore your sex drive, sexual desire, sexual arousal and libido. All the points, methods, techniques, foods, vitamins and minerals outlined in this book are not quick fix. Maintaining a healthy and mindful lifestyle and incorporating the foods, herbs and exercise discussed in this edition of the book, in your daily way of life should be a primary focus. The understanding that it is a continuous course of duty and lifestyle will make the intake of these food, herbs, vitamins and minerals to be effective in increasing and maintaining your sexual health. You need to pay attention to all points discussed in this book. When you lose your sex drive and libido, it also affects your sex partner and tolls on him/her, and he/she may start to look for an escape to the boredom – bedroom boredom. Good news is that there is therapy for the situation and you can be your own therapist, by just incorporating a healthy lifestyle aimed at improving your sex drive and your general health and well-being.

This guide tells you how.

PART 1

CHAPTER 1

HOW LONG SHOULD A NORMAL SEXUAL INTERCOURSE LAST?

First and foremost, the perfect duration of a normal sex is dependent on if you and your partner are satisfied at the end of every sex session irrespective of the duration of the intercourse. Living up to the popular expectations, up to the Johnsons is not normal. The length of a normal sex therefore is to the perception of the involved.

The media - TV, Radio, internet sites, sex columns, sex magazines and advent of Supper Sex Drugs has over the years created a "common understanding" of what the duration of sex should and should not be. Furthermore, it has created "genre of couples" with heightened preoccupation that they don't measure up, believing that they don't have sex often enough, sustain erections long enough and or last long enough when coupled and into back and forth thrusting before spitting and surrender. Some couples may even wonder if their orgasm is intense enough to measure to what they watched in sex movies, hear over the TV, Radio, read in sex columns and or what the super sex drugs promised on their labels. And most people believe that to have adequate and long enough erection and sex, one need a Viagra-like substance, drug or magic. Well, it is NOT so.

However, as said in the first few lines of this page: "...if you and your partner are satisfied..." the satisfaction must be real, not imaginary and or an attempt to be content with what is obtainable. Without doubt, every healthy adult should know the difference between what is normal and sub-normal. Of course we all know that there are categories of sexual intercourse including: quickie, normal sex, premature ejaculation, normal duration ejaculation.

Through research, timing and interview with people of different race, cultures, countries and continents, we established that average sex duration is between 3 minutes to 8 minutes, excluding the time spent in cuddling, seduction, foreplay and the actual

intercourse. In rare cases people can extend their duration to 14 minutes, once again excluding cuddling, seduction and foreplay. Discounting culture and religion, it is established that the average duration of sex including seduction, cuddling, foreplay and the actual intercourse is in the range of 30minutes to 45minutes.

A quickie and or premature ejaculation therefore could be said to be any sexual intercourse and or ejaculation under 3minutes.

Participants in our interviews and of timed sex sessions confessed that reaching the upper limits of the average duration of sex is aided by changing positions, practicing the use of love muscles to hold back the urge to surrender to quick orgasm and or cessation of thrusting movement while busy caressing, kissing, and or body sniffing.

Therefore, the average duration of sexual intercourse for normal people is anything between 3minutes to 8minutes and up to 14minutes for top tier sex candidates. While anything between 30minutes to 45minutes including cuddling, seduction, foreplay and sexual intercourse is the average duration of normal sex.

It is important to note that the above mentioned average times are only for the first session of sex. The second session with the same sex partner after some time elapses from the first session is often longer for all people.

What make some people last longer than others may have all to do with factors including:

✓ Health
✓ Style
✓ Tactic
✓ Experience
✓ Sexual attention span
✓ Sensual wiring
✓ Intensity of affection
✓ Mood

And more

Note: All stated under this topic "How Long Should a Normal Sexual Intercourse Last?" is with the assumption that the sex is not drug enhanced and or influenced – Drug free sex.

BL

CHAPTER 2

WHAT IS NORMAL SEX DRIVE (LIBIDO)?

Just like the question: how long should a normal sexual intercourse last?

There is no determination, measure or standard of a healthy or optimum level of sex drive or libido.

Sex drive is a person's desire for sex or a person's desire for sexual activity. Lack or loss of sexual desire can have a very negative impact on a relationship.

It is good to know that engaging in sexual activity and or intercourse does not in itself mean having a desire or sex drive. Some people may be having sex without a real desire, in which case they may be compelled to engage in sexual intercourse by their partner.

Sex drive or the desire to have sex integrates the body, the mind, the spirit, your entire sensuality. The physical erection of the penis on provocation in the case of a man, and the mere lying down and opening up to penetration and probably enjoying the act as it goes on, does not in itself constitute sex drive.

Sex drive is rather when your body, your mind and your spirit craves the ecstasy of sex including cuddling, seduction, foreplay, penetration intercourse and orgasm: intense orgasm with the attendant physical and emotional release, and surrender to the cellular level of the entire body system.

Sex drive therefore is inherent instinct and has components that are delicately interwoven and connected since birth. Such components integrate intricacies including emotion, sensuality, the spirit, the body, and ecstatic desires.

Sometimes, the connectivity of the intricate components of sex drive may be down and or not functioning optimally and that brings about low sex drive or sub-normal libido. In some cases, the connectivity of the intricate components of libido may enter into over-drive and lead to abnormal sex drive - hypersexuality. It is also good to know that erectile dysfunction (ED) does not represent low sex drive. The reason is that you may have the desire for sexual activity but have penile erectile dysfunction, which is a separate problem that requires a different kind of cure and or therapy. A person's sex drive may also vary from time to time depending on circumstances.

***** *****

FACTORS THAT INFLUENCE SEX DRIVE

- ➢ Biological Factors
- ➢ Psychological Factors
- ➢ Social Factors
- ➢ Physical Factors Or Exercise
- ➢ Sexual Dysfunction: - Sexual Desire Disorder, Sexual Arousal Disorder, Orgasm Disorder

➢ Medication

➢ Lifestyle

➢ Sexuality – Latent Homosexuality, Asexuality

➢ Health or Medical Condition

➢ Environmental and Climatic Factors

The factors and or components of an individual's sex drive may lead to low, normal or elevated sex drive of the individual.

This brings two questions up:

❖ What Causes Low Sex Drive?

❖ How to Improve or Revive Sex Drive?

In answering the two questions, we have to look into the individual factors and components of sex drive.

***** *****

BIOLOGICAL FACTORS AFFECTING SEX DRIVE

Hormonal level in the body system is one of the primary factors influencing a person's sex drive. The hormones in play as regards sex drive include:

Testosterone

Estrogen

Progesterone

TESTOSTERONE

Testosterone is sometimes called the "libido hormone" or "sex drive hormone". Its level in the body system affects both male and female sex drive. Optimal testosterone level in the body will give optimal sex drive. Testosterone may also boost your general energy level. More of testosterone will be discussed within the pages of this book. A woman's sex drive is highest sometime in the menstrual cycle, few days before ovulation and that is when she has the highest testosterone level in her body system. Also, the thickening of the uterine lining during the last days stimulates nerve endings making a woman to feel highly aroused. Testosterone level in men decreases with age. Testosterone is the single most culpable factor for low and or high sex drive in both males and females.

PROGESTERONE

Inadequate and or unwarranted high levels of progesterone causes low sex drive in women. In general, a balance is needed between the hormones for an optimal sex drive. Improving low progesterone level to the optimal levels improves one's sex drive. Women have used the application of progesterone cream to revive their libido. Progesterone is also one of the dominant hormones at ovulation when a woman is most fertile. Normally progesterone level is more in men than in women. It is more a male than a female hormone.

ESTROGEN

Decrease in estrogen level and its associated vaginal dryness, painful sexual intercourse may cause low sex drive in women. Menopausal women generally have decreased estrogen level and low sex drive.

Normal level of estrogen in female is healthy for normal sex desire. High estrogen levels in men leads to a situation called estrogen dominance and this causes low sex drive among other sexual related problems.

An excessive Estrogen level in the body is called <u>Estrogen Dominance</u>.

How Estrogen Dominance in Men Affects Sex Drive/Libido?

Estrogen dominance is the term used to represent the state of hormonal imbalance of more than normal levels of estrogen in the body system. Estrogen dominance is more common in women than men, it can also affect men.

The adverse effect of estrogen dominance is more potent in men than in women.

In men estrogen dominance causes a range of problems including low sex drive or diminished libido, infertility, erectile dysfunction, enlarged prostate, and certain types of cancer.

Estrogen for the most part is a female hormone. However, it is also naturally produced by the male body in relatively small quantity. Hormonal imbalance caused by estrogen dominance (more than normal level) is a hormone imbalance that occurs when levels of the hormone estrogen are too high in relation to other hormones in the body such as testosterone and progesterone. However, estrogen dominance may also occur when the body for some reason secretes excessive levels of estrogen into the system. It may also occur due to under-secretion of other sex hormones like progesterone and testosterone.

Other Serious Causes of Estrogen Dominance Include:

Alcoholism

Obesity

Xenoestrogens – exposure to environmental estrogen

Pituitary glands malfunction (Pituitary Disease)

Testicular Tumors

Prostate Disease

Symptoms of Estrogen Dominance or Excessive Estrogen Levels in Men

- Diminished Libido or Low sex drive
- Erectile dysfunction
- Infertility
- Gynecomastia (enlarged male breast or man boobs)
- Overweight, Weight Gain, Obesity
- Enlarged prostate or Prostate Cancer
- Testicular Cancer

How to Avoid Estrogen Dominance

Healthy Weight

Estrogen is produced by fat cells, it is produced from cholesterols. Obese individuals have lots of cholesterol and other fatty cells in their body, creating a healthy laboratory for the production of estrogen and creating hormonal imbalance that is an enemy of healthy libido/sex drive in both men and women.

Hydration

Stay adequately hydrated to optimize the functions of the kidney. Optimal kidney function is necessary for the body hormonal balance. About 5 – 8 glasses of water daily is not bad.

Eat Fiber Rich Foods

Eating food rich in dietary fiber will help reduce excessive estrogen in the body by binding to the estrogen and removing them from the body as waste. Dietary fiber is also known to prevent colon cancer and prevents constipation. Constipation worsens estrogen dominance.

Exercise

Regular exercise promotes healthy hormone balance.

Abstain From Alcohol as Much as Possible

Alcohol stimulates the body to produce more estrogen. Alcohol also interferes with the normal or proper functioning of the kidneys especially its ability to filter off excessive estrogen from the body system. Alcoholism is one of the major causes of estrogen dominance in men. Alcoholic men never have good libido/sex drive.

Avoid Exposure to Xenoestrogens

Xenoestrogens are manufactured substances by man called endocrine disruptors. These substances which are present in products ranging from beauty products (nail polish), dairy products, foods, meat, plastic products, laundry detergents, chemical pesticides and herbicides used in the farms to grow fruits and vegetables. The meat, dairy products and poultry pick up these substances from the growth hormones and other substances used to raise the animals in the farms.

The substances have estrogen-like activities in the body, in that they mimic the activities of estrogen in the body just like phytoestrogens.

Avoidance

Remove cling wraps from meats and other foods when you get home from the grocery stores. Cling wraps used in covering these foods contains DHEA, an estrogenic substance

Do not microwave foods with cling wrap or plastic

Minimize eating canned or tinned foods as the lining contains BPA which is a proud and known xenoestrogen that leaks into food when exposed to heat.

EFFECTS OF EXCESSIVE ESTROGEN IN THE BODY

Low/Diminished Libido

Depression

Low Zinc in the body – (not good for sex drive)

High Copper retention by the body – (not good for sex drive, normal retention is necessary)

Erectile dysfunction/impotence (in men)

Prostate problems (men)

Thyroid malfunction

Depressed levels of progesterone

Endometriosis

Breast cancer

Fatigue

Mood swings

Water-retention/bloating

Dry skin

PSYCHOLOGICAL FACTORS AFFECTING SEX DRIVE

Psychological injuries and issues such as experience of sexual abuse, assault, trauma, or neglect, body image issues, sexual performance, vaginal dryness, vaginal health, loose vagina, distraction or depression may affect libido of both males and females. Other factors may include lack of privacy, lack of intimacy, unresolved relationship problems.

Female who are victims of sex abuse such as rape at a young age and or any age may develop low libido as a result. Sexual abuse, sexual assault of all sorts and at all age may bring about lack of interest in sex and low sex drive.

Neglect of a person by peers, husband, and friends may bring about low self-esteem and low sex drive.

Perception of self-body image may be a factor of low sex drive.

The believe that one does not have an adequate performance on bed during sexual intercourse may lead to low sex drive as the victim tries to recluse to self to avoid embarrassment and disappointment.

Vaginal dryness which causes severe pain during intercourse may contribute to low sex drive. General vaginal health including vaginal odor may also be a deterrent to vibrant sex drive.

Depression is a big determinant of sex drive. When people are depressed, sex drive is relegated to the back bench.

Lack of privacy may also affect someone's sex drive.

Unresolved relationship problems of all sorts may also be a source of low sex drive.

In general, low sex drive caused by psychological factors may be cured and corrected by reconnecting your psychological self with one's physical, spiritual and sensuality.

Remember, Sex drive is when your body, your mind and your spirit craves the ecstasy of sex including cuddling, seduction, foreplay, penetration, intercourse and orgasm: intense orgasm with the attendant physical and emotional release, and surrender to the cellular level of the entire body system. Sex drive therefore is an inherent instinct and has components that are delicately interwoven and connected since birth.

The said components integrate intricacies including emotion, sensuality, the spirit, the body, and ecstatic desires. Low sex drive of psychological source may be rebooted by merely reviving the connectivity of the said intricate components.

Reconnecting your psychological being to the intricate components of sex drive may involve resolving the source of the psychological injury as a single and separate cure, or therapy.

Sexual abuse and assault may be resolved by seeing a sex therapist, and or psychologist.

Neglect may be resolved by reaching out, to see who is neglecting who.

Unresolved relationship issues should be resolved by reaching out to your partner for talks and open communication.

Body image issues may be resolved by lifestyle solutions.

Vaginal dryness, vaginal health and loose vagina – see the book The Bedroom Fool: Vaginal Tightening and Rejuvenation.

SOCIAL FACTORS AFFECTING LOW SEX DRIVE

Social factors such as work and family related problems may be sources of low sex drive.

PHYSICAL FACTORS/EXERCISE AND SEX DRIVE

Adequate and or lack of exercise can influence the sex drive of an individual. The fitness level and feeling good improves the physiological functions of the body. Exercise makes people feel good about themselves and feeling good about oneself is a prelude to a healthy sex drive. Being fit may lead to optimum sexual performance which boosts drive for comeback/repeat encounter. And sex in itself is exercise of sort and requires strength, endurance and fitness.

During and after exercise the body releases hormones such as testosterone, adrenalin and endorphins in the blood stream. The combination of these hormones produces the feel good and wellbeing mood. It is so true in both males and females that people who engage in regular exercise craves it, and become somewhat deprived or unhappy and grumpy when they stop and or couldn't exercise.

However, it is good to know that too much exercise may lead to low sex drive as it may lead to cessation of the production of the feel good hormones and increase the presence of the stress hormone - cortisol. Stress is sex drive inhibitor -killer.

TYPES OF EXERCISE AND THEIR SPECIFIC EFFECTS

YOGA

Yoga practice increases sensitivity and stimulates the flow of blood to the pelvis, the pelvic floor muscles, and the genitals. Adequate and steady blood flow to the pelvic floor muscles and the genital is a star sex drive factor. Yoga has also been said to improve the intensity of orgasm. Some yoga positions are said to tone genital muscles.

POPULAR YOGA POSITIONS
  - ➢ The Camel Position

➢ The upward-facing Position

➢ Dog Position

➢ The Butterfly Position

WEIGHT LIFTING EXERCISE

Lifting small to medium weights of dumbbells may help in the release of endorphin, testosterone and adrenalin. Weight lifting may bring about improved bone density and stronger muscles.

***** *****

***** *****

SEXUAL DESIRE DISORDER

SEXUAL DYSFUNCTION

SEXUAL MALFUNCTION

Any difficulty arising during any phase or stage of a normal sexual activity is referred to as sexual dysfunction or sexual malfunction. Such difficulty includes:

❖ Sexual Desire Disorder

❖ Sexual Arousal Disorder

❖ Orgasm Disorder - Anorgasmia

Sexual Desire Disorder

Sexual desire disorders sometimes called decreased libido is the absence and or lack of desire for sex, sexual activity, sexual or erotic imagination and fantasies. This may be lack or diminished desire for a particular ones sex partner and or general decreased sexual desire. For a disorder to be qualified as sexual desire disorder, the victim's sexual desire must have been normal and healthy in the past or the victim's sexual desire have always been low or no desire at all.

Sexual desire disorder may be caused by any of the following:

Hormonal Imbalance

Hormonal imbalance such as sudden decrease in estrogen level in a woman's body system and or decrease in man's testosterone level is one of the causes of sexual desire disorder. Decrease in normal level of testosterone in a woman's system may also cause sexual desire disorder.

Aging

Aging is always a culprit when it comes to decrease in hormonal levels and proper functioning of the body system. As we age every function in the body system ages along leading to certain defects and disorders

Fatigue

Lack of energy in itself is a sign of one imbalance or the other in the system.

Pregnancy

Pregnancy entails lots of changes in the body, including hormonal changes.

Medication

Medication may induce over production, secretion of a particular hormone and or other biochemical such as enzymes in the body system. The said production or secretion may bring about imbalance of sorts.

Depression and Anxiety

Both can also be culprits in sexual desire dysfunction

Sexual Arousal Disorders

In men, sexual arousal dysfunction is better known as <u>Erectile Dysfunction</u> (sometimes wrongly referred to as impotence). In women sexual arousal dysfunction is referred to as <u>Frigidity</u>.

ERECTILE DYSFUNCTION

It is good to note that erectile dysfunction in itself in not lack of sexual desire. A person who suffers from erectile dysfunction may have sexual desire, sexual fantasies and erotic fantasies, but may not be able to have and sustain erection.

Erectile dysfunction is the inability of a sexually matured man to have and sustain an erection of the penis or penile erection.

Causes of Erectile Dysfunction include:

Damaged or Malfunction of the Nervi Eregentis

Nervi erigentes also called Pelvic splanchnic nerves starts from the sacral spinal nerves S2 - S4. From here, they contribute to the innervation/blood supply of the pelvic and genital organs, supplying the capillaries in the region. This nerve is responsible for lifting up or erecting the penis when engorged with blood. The nerve is also responsible for emptying of the urinary bladder and rectum. It therefore makes some sense saying that someone with erectile dysfunction may possibly have some form of urinary and defecation malfunction. A damaged nervi eregentis may prevent erection entirely, whereas, a dysfunctional nervi eregentis delays erection and or do not sustain an erection long enough. However this condition is reversible.

Diabetes

Diabetes may cause a reduction in the supply of blood to the nervi erigentes and the genital capillaries. Diabetes is reversible.

FRIGIDITY

There may be medical causes to this disorder, including decreased blood flow to the female genitals, the pelvic floor muscles or lack of vaginal lubrication.

For more information on this topic see the book

The Bedroom Fool.

***** *****

***** *****

ORGASM DISORDER OR ANORGASMIA

This disorder is called delayed ejaculation in males. Anorgasmia or orgasm disorder is a condition when an individual takes too long to reach and or achieve orgasm or unable to reach and or achieve orgasm even with maximum stimulation. This situation is more common in females than males. This condition may lead to sexual frustration and eventually lack of interest in sex- low sex drive. The statistics as at the year 2008 shows that about 15% of women have difficulties with orgasm, and 10% of women in the United States alone have never climaxed/had orgasm.

And only 29% of women have had and always have orgasms with their partner during sexual intercourse. While orgasm with men diminished as they age. Women are more likely to understand and achieve regular orgasm as they age.

Causes of Orgasm disorder include:

- ✓ The use of antidepressants
- ✓ Psychiatric disorder
- ✓ Diabetic neuropathy
- ✓ Multiple sclerosis
- ✓ Genital mutilation
- ✓ Surgery
- ✓ Pelvic trauma – from wounds in the pelvic region
- ✓ Hormonal Imbalance
- ✓ Hysterectomy
- ✓ Spinal cord Injury
- ✓ Drug (opiate) addiction

Causes of anorgasmia (orgasm disorder) differ with type of anorgasmia.

TYPES OF ANORGASMIA

Primary Anorgasmia

A person with primary anorgasmia has never experienced orgasm. Primary anorgasmia is more prevalent in women than in men.

This type of anorgasmia occurs in men who do not have bulb-cavernous reflex. Women victims of primary anorgasmia are not easily aroused sexually, and receive very little sexual excitement. Due to lack of release of orgasmic energy after stimulation and engorgement of the genitals, they often suffer from sexual frustration, restlessness, and pelvic pain.

Sexual repression due to culture and or religion has been touted as possible causes of women primary anorgasmia.

Male primary anorgasmia may be caused by circumcision. As men get older, the ability to reach orgasm diminishes. Remember the mere fact that a man ejaculates does not mean he reached or achieved orgasm.

Secondary Anorgasmia

A person suffering from secondary anorgasmia is a person who have been having orgasm but for one reason or the other losses the ability to achieve orgasm over time.

Men and women have about equal chances of suffering from secondary anorgasmia.

Causes of secondary anorgasmia include:

- ➢ Alcoholism
- ➢ Depression
- ➢ Grief
- ➢ Surgery – Chiefly hysterectomy
- ➢ Vaginal reconstructive Surgery (vaginaplasty)
- ➢ Decrease or lack of Estrogen (in women)

➤ Psychological injury and trauma such as "rape"

➤ Prostate cancer and prostatectomy

Situational Anorgasmia:

This is a situation whereby a person achieves orgasm in one situation and not in another. The situation may be the type of sexual stimulation, different partners, certain conditions, duration and intensity of foreplay.

Random Anorgasmia

This is a situation where one has not have orgasm enough on a regular or near regular basis to be able to establish the desirability of orgasm.

TREATMENT

Erectile Dysfunction could be treated among other treatments with penis pump. Sialidase (an enzyme) as well as Yohimbine hydrochloride is being touted as viable in treating damaged or mal functioning nerves such as nervi eregentis. This is because yohimbe extract or yohimbine chloride is a very potent aphrodisiac.

Lifestyle Changes such as stop smoking and abandoning alcoholism can be very helpful.

Yohimbine is the main active chemical ingredient (an alkaloid) from the bark of the West African evergreen tree with scientific name Pausinystalia Yohimbe formerly known as corynanthe yohimbe from the Rubiaceae family of the plant kingdom. Yohimbe tree is found in West Africa including Southwestern Nigeria, Gabon, and Cameroun. The tree also grows in eastern Africa, in Zaire. About 31 other alkaloids are present in the bark of the Yohimbe tree. In Africa and around the world, yohimbe is used as an aphrodisiac. Yohimbine hydrochloride is the manufactured standard form of Yohimbine. Yohimbine is effective for the treatment of erectile dysfunction, and for low sex drive/libido in women. Other plants with similar alkaloids are Rauwolfia Serpentina (Indian Snakeroot) and Alchornea floribunda (Niando).

Yohimbine has been touted for the treatment of type 2 diabetes.

Female Sexual Dysfunctions as discussed above could be treated using:

Hormonal patches – to correct hormonal imbalance

Hormonal tablets – to correct hormonal imbalance

Clitoral vacuum pump – to improve blood flow to the clitoris, genitals, improve sensation, improve sexual arousal

Sexual Pain Disorders: Sexual pain disorder is sometimes called Vaginismus. This is the involuntary contraction of the vaginal muscles leading to the closure of the opening of the vagina, making any type of penetration difficult and painful. See the Book "The Bedroom Fool" for more information.

Hypoactive Sexual Desire Disorder (HSDD)
OR Sexual Aversion Disorder

This is the lack and or absence of erotic desire, sexual desire, sexual fantasy and or lack of interest in sexual activity. This disorder must have resulted to distress and interpersonal frictions to be classified as HSDD. This disorder may manifest in forms such as: general lack of or diminished sexual desire, lack of sexual desire for an existing partner, lack of sexual desire after a life of normal sexual desire, and lack or diminished sexual desire since birth.

Medication and Sex Drive

Being on certain medication may induce over production, secretion of a particular hormone and or other biochemical such as enzymes in the body system. The said production or secretion may bring about imbalance of sorts. Medication may also lead to depression and anxiety Hormonal and chemical imbalance in the body, depression and anxiety may lead to decreased libido.

Lifestyle and Sex Drive

Lifestyles that may affect libido include:

Smoking – smoking decreases libido

Alcoholism – alcoholism decreases libido

Exercise – regular normal exercise improves libido

Diet and Nutrition – some food have direct effect on libido

Weight - Overweight or Underweight

Stressful Life (Stress) – stress inhibits libido

LATENT HOMOSEXUALITY

Latent homosexuality is an erotic desire or sexual desire towards members of the same sex. However, the said desire or inclination is never consciously expressed in any form or manner. It is therefore a hidden, repressed and or unrecognized sexuality which is most unlikely be explored. Most often, the person who has latent homosexuality do not know which may be the reason why it is never expressed. This may bring about low sex drive. The phrase latent homosexuality is first coined by Sigmund Freud.

ASEXUALITY

Asexuality is the lack of sexual attraction towards other people irrespective of gender. It is also lack of interest in sex, or lack of sexual orientation. Asexual individuals have little or no sex drive.

HEALTH AND SEX DRIVE

Health of an individual including vaginal health may affect the sex drive of the individual. For information on vaginal health such as vaginal dryness, vaginal prolapse, Loose Vagina, see the book:

"The Bedroom Fool" by Be Your Dream Press.

BL

CHAPTER 3

SEXUAL ADDICTION

Sexual addiction is the term used to explain and or identify sexual urges, sexual outbursts, sexual behaviors, sexual thoughts that occur extremely frequently in an individual and often out of control of the individual.

Terms used to identify different sex addictions include:

Hypersexuality

Sexual Compulsivity

Sexual Impulsivity

Excessive Sexual drive

Satyriasis – (males)

Nymphomania (females)

Persistent Genital Arousal Disorder (PGAD)

Persistent Sexual Arousal Syndrome (PSAS)

Persistent Genital Arousal Syndrome (PGAS)

Hypersexuality/Nymphomania/Sexual Compulsivity/Satyriasis

This type of sex addiction is often associated with diminished sexual inhibition. Diminished sexual inhibition may cause extremely frequent or suddenly increased sexual urge, often out of control of the individual.

Causes May Include:

Unknown

Medical Conditions

Biochemical or Physiological changes associated with Dementia

Persistent Sexual (Genital) Arousal Disorder/Syndrome

This is a condition where a female's genital is spontaneously, persistently, and uncontrollably aroused with or without engorgement, sexual desire and or orgasm. This may persist for hours days and or weeks. Orgasm may sometimes provide temporary relief to the symptom, however, the symptom returns with hours and or the next day. It may affect people at any age. It has been said to be caused by irregular function of some sensory nerves and or in premenopausal women or postmenopausal women who underwent hormonal treatment.

Sex addiction in all its types and identifications have not been catalogued by the Diagnostic and Statistical Manual of Mental Disorder IV (DSM – IV). And no real/sustainable cure and or treatment have been established.

PART 2

REMEDIES TO LOW SEX DRIVE / LOW LIBIDO

HOW TO AWAKEN, IMPROVE, AND REVIVE SEX DRIVE

BL

CHAPTER 4

HOW TO AWAKEN SEX DRIVE

CONTRARY TO POPULAR BELIEF, DECREASED SEX DRIVE (Libido)

Is <u>Not An Inevitable Consequence of Aging.</u>

SEX DRIVE (Libido) IS AN INSTINCT

Libido is inherent to humans. Sometimes it is at its normal energetic level (during certain ages of life) or it may lie low (sleeping) and needs some awakening. And at other times it may be bruised and needs some revival or it may be dead/damaged and needs to be remedied. Notwithstanding the state of the human sex drive, it is always possible to rekindle libido.

Yes You Can Still Have Sex Again in this Lifetime!

For the purpose of this chapter, let's divide Sex Drive into three Components:

- ❖ Imagination/Fantasy/Dream
- ❖ Urge – Renewable inherent energy encased in the subconscious
- ❖ Sex and Orgasm - Release and surrender of the renewable energy

The imagination, fantasy or dream is driven and directed by the trapped inherent renewable subconscious sexual energy. The urge to reach out for the physical contact or consummation of the fantasy/imagination is driven by hormones.

The awakening of this energy to drive the imagination, fantasy or desire is the process of bringing it up from the subconscious to the conscious level, and the process differs from one individual to another.

The process is always as diverse as the cause of the 'sleep', which may range from emotional, psychological, physical, etc., as discussed in the previous chapter under causes of low libido.

Remember, the energy of sex, the energy of sexual desire and attraction to the opposite sex is not an ordinary or banal energy. It is the energy of the continuity of life, and in this case the energy that is an integral component of the alchemy, the chemistry of the continuity of human existence.

And this energy is alive throughout life even when what we know within the realms of biological possibility points to the contrary. It could be awakened and revived at any point of human life.

At a certain stage in life, one wouldn't necessarily need to have sex with another human being (sexual intercourse) to be and feel sexed. At that and such points, it is not so much as having interest in physical sexual intercourse as in being able to articulate the entire sexual energy, including erotic energy, nervous system energy, the endocrine system energy, sensory system energy, the lymphatic system energy, the digestive system energy, visual energy, emotional energy into that awakening and enlightening pull.

It is just very true that nothing awakens and enlightens the brain and the entire body system more than the pull of sexual attraction and desire.

To have a smooth and effective reawakening of sex drive, we need to dissect sex into its entire component and then identify the part(s) that most turns us on. And once you identify what is your softest spot of sex and sexual desire, then you can conveniently work on it, to unleash the energy.

In working on the most erotic stimuli of your sexual imagination and fantasy, you must surrender, and block away all and any inhibition that may block your freedom of imagination and fantasy.

DISSECTING SEX

FIND OUT WHAT YOU REALLY LOVE ABOUT IT AND AWAKEN IT

SIGHT OR VISUALS

Visualizing/seeing a potential sex partner is the first step and feeling you endure of sexual attraction. Even in your imagination and dreams of sexual fantasy, there is always a picture of the type of sexual partner that is interwoven into your psyche of what an attractive partner should look like. The magic of visual conception and fascination is an integral part of sex drive and sexual energy.

To awaken your sex drive, you need to rekindle this pictorial imagination/fantasy by visiting and or positioning yourself where it is most likely to see your type (physical) of partners. You may need to visit places for this purpose. The beaches, downtown, parks, gardens, movie theaters, rallies, concerts, etc., are good places to start.

SOUND

There are sounds associated with some intimate and romantic moments of your sexual life. Sounds that make your sex drive boom and boost. Such sounds form part of the entire sexual desire and drive. Reintegrating yourself with such sounds will add a positive forward step to the awakening process of your sex drive.

Sounds Such As:

- ✓ Music
- ✓ Melody
- ✓ Singing birds
- ✓ Roaring tide
- ✓ Stream
- ✓ The creek
- ✓ Moaning
- ✓ Laughter
- ✓ Wind

ENVIRONMENT/PLACE

Some types of environment and place evoke sexual desire in people. It may be some quiet place in the woods, by the banks of a lonely and quiet river/creek, the beach, the theater, sand-dooms, mountain, valleys, hilly country side, the sea, etc.

TOUCHING

Touch for the most part could be erotic and stirs sexual desire. If touching is one of the acts that stir your sex drive, then you need to employ it. The touching could be massage by a professional masseur or touching from your sex partner. Whichever one that floats your boat is the one you need to employ.

ODOR

The sense of smell is naturally very closely associated with romance, sex drive, sexual desire and sex of the animal kingdom. This makes me remember the he/male goat.

The smell emitted by the opposite sex is a great turn on, sexually. You may need to obtain some human pheromones that are available in the cosmetic and perfume stores. Provided the sensory receptors in the vomeronasal of the olfactory lobes are healthy, they will transmit the message to the frontal lobe of the brain for processing, and probably ignite/awaken sexual desire.

Pheromones? What is Pheromones?

Pheromones are chemicals that can act, radiate, emit from the body of the secreting/emitting individual to influence the behavior of the receiving individual of the same species.

Men release pheromones in their sweat mainly the armpit sweat. Women release their pheromones when they become fertile. The sensory receptors in the olfactory lobes detect the pheromones and send the message to the hypothalamus of the brain for processing. The message triggers sexual desire and attraction in both sexes. Positive response and invitation depends on the strength of the pheromones and how much the receiving individual is smitten.

TASTE

Taste is an integral part of the sensory system, and plays a role in awakening sex drive and or sexual desire. Some people's sexual desire and or drive may be associated with a particular taste. It may be taste of food, fruit, drink and or the taste of kissing.

You know more than anybody else what floats your boat. Employ it to your sex drive awakening process.

STORIES: Nothing creates and revives imagination and fantasies more than stories. Such stories include: Printed Stories with images and pictures- Pictorials, Sex magazines

Printed stories – romance novels

Visual Stories – Movies, sex films

If this is what floats your sexual imagination boat, then indulge in it.

In doing all that is outlined in this section of the book, you need not rush. You must continue with dissecting and re-dissecting sex until you find the real thing that floats your sexual imagination and fantasy. Once you find it or them, you must act on it until you start to have sexual imagination and fantasy again. Do not rush, it is therapy. Once you reawaken your imagination, and sexual fantasy, you are done with the stage.

At this point you have awakened the primary part of sex drive, which is sexual/erotic imagination and fantasy. The next step is to transform the imagination and fantasy into sexual desire.

BL

CHAPTER 5

DISSECT AND REVIEW YOUR LIFE

In the last chapter, we dissected sex and identified what you actually like most about sex, and have you work on them to awaken your libido. Now, it is only reasonable if we pay attention to the fingers that are pointing back at you while you were pointing the accusing/dissecting finger at sex. We will now have you review your life to see if there is anything within, that may be as much a culprit. What is your daily schedule including from the time you wake up, to the breakfast table, to leaving for work through coming back home to going back to sleep at bed time.

Make a detailed list of it, leaving nothing behind. Do you have enough rest/break time in-between your daily shores?

Remember, the body needs consistent break time and rest to restore and replenish energy, minerals and hormones for proper functioning. When the body does not receive enough rest it is stressed out and the stress will start to accumulate in the system - big enemy of libido. Do you have enough sleep in every 24 hour cycle of the day?

Nothing substitutes sleep, not even rest. Enough sleep is a must for the proper and optimal functioning of all the body system including the nervous system, the endocrine system, the brain, and sensory system, the immune system, reproductive system, and the circulatory system. Any and all the system of the body is directly or indirectly dependent on sleep for replenishment.

Remedy is Simple – Make out more time for relaxation, rest and sleep. You need at least seven hours sleep every 24hours cycle. Of the 7 hour sleep time, 6 hours must be straight sleep preferably during night time. The remaining one hour could be shared between naps during normal daily activity.

No matter how busy you are, you can achieve the 7-hr minimum sleep time every 24hr cycle if you employ proper time management for your schedule.

Time-Management

Allot time and limit to all and every of your daily activity. Make out time for rest/break between activities. Make out time for naps between activities. Manage your time adequately, and do not over work yourself.

HOW SLEEP AFFECTS YOUR LIBIDO

Sleep is an elevated restful and anabolic state. During sleep, revival, growth and rejuvenation of the immune, nervous, reproductive, skeletal and muscular systems takes place. It is very important to most members of the animal kingdom including all mammals, all birds, many reptiles, amphibians, and fish.

Chemicals called *neurotransmitters* control sleep or wakefulness by acting on different groups of nerve cells, or neurons, in the brain. Neurons in the brainstem, which connects the brain with the spinal cord, produce neurotransmitters such as serotonin and norepinephrine. Serotonin and Norepinephrine keep some parts of the brain active while we are awake. A chemical called adenosine accumulates in the blood while we are awake and causes drowsiness if we stay too long without sleep. This chemical gradually breaks down while we sleep. Neurons that control sleep interact closely with the immune system. Decreased serotonin levels can lead to chronic fatigue, sleep disorders and changes in appetite. Fatigue is an enemy of healthy sex drive.

Human Growth Hormone (HGH) is replenished and its level in the body system rises during deep sleep. The human body relies on chemical components to maintain a constant state of balance. This state of balance is called homeostasis. When one or more of the body chemicals fall out of balance due to increase or decrease in their levels, this may cause the systems of the body to work less efficiently. Chemical imbalances in the reproductive system can cause infertility and low Sex Drive in both men and women. Low levels of estrogen and testosterone can affect sex drive, sexual desire and sexual performance.

Develop High Self-Esteem

Strong and high self-esteem breeds feel good state of mind. Feeling good and high self-esteem accentuates sensuality and boost sexual drive and sexual desire. Low self-esteem may be due to dissatisfaction with one's appearance including body weight, structure and or shape. This may be due to standard created by media and society. Dissatisfaction with oneself may cause depression and anxiety; both are known enemies of healthy sex drive and libido. This is a growing problem among North American women as noted by the American Psychological Association, in stating that 30-40% of women are somewhat not satisfied and unhappy with their appearance, and 45% of women develop symptoms of anxiety or depression associated with dissatisfaction with their appearance. It is good to know that beauty is in the eye of the beholder, and you can find your own standard and definition of beauty. Focus on you and maintaining good health. Surrounding yourself with good people and positive thinkers is a good way to go.

Have fun and celebrate life in ways that will accentuate your happiness and health including: running, dancing, cycling, traveling, breathing, laughing, dreaming, mediation, fantasizing, etc.

BL

CHAPTER 6

TRANSFORM YOUR EROTIC OR SEXUAL IMAGINATION AND FANTASY INTO SEXUAL DESIRE AND SEXUAL AROUSAL

Now that the sexual imagination and fantasy have been awakened through dissecting sex and identifying what turns you on the most, the mind has been awakened and the brain stimulated. The cerebral cortex of the frontal lobe of the brain is the origin of command for the production of physical stimuli – the hormones that drive sexual desire, arousal or urge. The sexual desire and or arousal will be revived in anticipation for sexual activity. At this metamorphic stage of your sexuality and sensuality, you need to reconnect your physical self with the physical erotic stimuli and the sexual imagination. In so doing, you will learn if the sexual imagination and the physical stimuli bring sexual desire and sexual arousal.

Furthermore, you will also learn if the desire and or arousal lead to penile erection in case of men or genital engorgement, vaginal lubrication and in some cases nipples hardening in case of women.

Remember, as said in the earlier chapters, sex drive is an instinct driven by sexual energy. The energy is encased in the subconscious and the process of awakening your sexual imagination, and transferring it from the mind to the brain, where physical stimuli that drives the energy from the brain through the spinal cord to the S2-S4 sacral spinal nerve is generated. The energy is delivered to the pelvic splanchnic nerves which start from the sacral spinal nerves S2 to S4. From here, the energy is dissipated and they contribute to the innervation/blood supply of the pelvic floor and genital organs, supplying the capillaries in the region.

If the above is established, then, you have lifted your sexual energy from the subconscious mind where it was encased to the conscious mind where it is at liberty to unleash.

So How Do We Know You Did All this?

PLAY WITH YOURSELF

Sounds odd, doesn't it? Somehow, yes. However, it does not really sound proper when playing with oneself becomes odd. In other words it is embarrassing in itself to know that people feel odd, shy and embarrassed when masturbation is brought up for discussion. Playing with oneself should not necessarily be for orgasm to be achieved. Really, it is more of sexual/circulatory/innervation exercise to make sure that blood supply and circulation to the genitals is healthy. Practicing this blood circulatory exercise to achieve arousal/erection or engorgement of the genitals is very healthy in itself and may preserve your sexual arousal health. Trying out with yourself is a way of improving the animal instinct of sexuality (sexual desire) in you, if possible increasing it many folds to bring the urge and sexual desire (sex drive) to the level where you will be grabbing or reaching out for the physical contact/consummation of your sexual fantasy/imagination, sexual desire with another human being. If that happens then you have completely reawakened, revived and or remedied your sex drive, your libido. Playing with yourself does not necessarily mean achieving or reaching orgasm, but, merely to see if you can get some arousal.

Remember, the whole process started because you have low or diminished sex drive, and you need to revive it. You are engaged in a therapy.

There is this misconception about masturbation.

Most people think masturbation is for people who don't have sex partners, but it is not true, at least for the purpose of this book, and this study.

Besides, if you don't know how to be sensual and sexual with yourself, if you do not know how to arouse yourself, then, how do you expect to be good at it with a partner? For the purpose of this section of the book, this therapy, you need to try it to see the connection you have made between your sexual fantasy, the erotic stimuli originating from the cerebral cortex of the frontal lobe of the brain and the physical you. Once the three links are connected, and established, your sex drive/libido is revived and you will then go on to the next stage which is sexual gratification - orgasm.

Tried it? Did you have erection? Vaginal Lubrication? Nipples Hardening?

Yes? Bingo!

No? ooh!

If you do not achieve erection, vaginal lubrication, or if you do have a minimal or weak erection, minimal lubrication, it means that the erotic physical stimuli provided by the hormones are weak and not enough to sustain the imagination and fantasy that have been awakened.

This will take us to Sex Drive Revival through remedies/therapy such as:

- ➢ Food
- ➢ Vitamins
- ➢ Minerals
- ➢ Aphrodisiacs
- ➢ Hormone Replacement
- ➢ Etc.

PART 3

FOODS:: HERBS:: VITAMINS:: MINERALS:: APHRODISIACS

AND HORMONES TO IMPROVE/REVIVE SEX DRIVE/LIBIDO

CHAPTER 7

FOODS AND FRUITS TO IMPROVE SEX DRIVE

The foods discussed in this section of the book may have some other health benefits. However, they are chosen for discussion based on their importance as regards mainly sex drive, libido and general reproductive health and benefits.

QUINOA

Quinoa is a native of Andean region of Bolivia, Ecuador, Columbia and Peru. It is a grain-like crop cultivated for its nutrient-rich seeds. It is a pseudo-cereal of the Chenopodium (goosefoot) specie from Chenopodioideae sub-family of the Amarenthaceae family of the plant kingdom.

Quinoa contains complete chain of vegetable protein with nine essential amino-acids including omega-3 fatty acids and particularly very high content of lysine. Quinoa is also high in its content of Zinc, B-vitamins, B6, B2, iron, Magnesium, Phosphorous, and Vitamin E.

Lysine is the building block/strands of elastin and elastin aids the production of collagen. Elastin is a structural protein responsible for the elastic nature of the connective tissues such as the skin, blood vessels, penis, vaginal walls and canal, Pc muscles, ligaments, lungs, joints, cartilages, etc.

Elastin or otherwise called tropoelastin is a structural protein responsible for elasticity (stretching, recovery or recoil) found mainly in connective tissues such as vaginal wall, the penis, skin, blood vessels (chiefly the aorta), joints, ligaments, cartilages. Elastin allows tissue to resume or return to their original shape/size after stretching or contracting. In this case, it helps the vagina to return to its original size after stretches such as in child-birth, insertion of large objects, and loosening and aids the penis to return to its normal size after stretching from excitement. In the human body, elastin is biochemically coded by the gene known as the ELN. Elastin is made up of randomly coiled fibers of about 830 essential amino acids that are cross-linked into a durable form, and lysine is chiefly responsible for the cross-linkage. The two types of links found in elastin are: desmosine link and isodesmosine link.

Remember the ridges or folds of the vaginal wall?

Elastin is responsible for the ridges (coils or folds).

Elastin is also found in the bladder and the lungs (expands when full of urine or air respectively and contracts when emptied).

Deficiency of elastin causes:

General loss of elasticity such as in blood vessels, Loose vagina, penis, Loose bladder (incontinence)

Emphysema (shortness of breath) as in the lungs, caused by alpha-1-antitrypsin deficiency

Marfan's Syndrome

Elastin therefore aids in the health of the blood vessels, as such it is very essential to adequate and proper blood circulation and supply. Proper blood circulation and supply is a primer to erection, sexual desire, sexual arousal, sex drive and libido.

Elastin maintains the health of the blood vessels surrounding the penis and is the building strands of the vaginal wall muscle fibers. Elastin and collagen works hand in hand and are oftentimes produced simultaneously. Both form the support for the suspension or connecting the vaginal canal to the pelvic floor. And both are replete in the skin around the penis and muscle strands of the penis.

The lysine content of quinoa is high. Lysine, or L-lysine, is an essential amino acid. The human body cannot produce or synthesize lysine.

Lysine restores and or promotes the production of arginine in the body system.

Lysine helps restore arginine to its normal levels. L-arginine promotes circulation and relaxes blood vessels. L-arginine is essential for the body production of nitric oxide. Nitric oxide helps to open the potassium channel, which causes the blood vessels to relax – vasodilation, and this aids the proper blood circulation and blood supply to the genitals. Adequate blood supply to the genitals aids sexual arousal, sexual desire, sex drive, and libido.

The body system produces its own L-arginine. However, L-lysine aids the arginine to reach its adequate and or optimum level in the body system.

L-arginine may also stimulate growth hormones, including testosterone which is the libido hormone.

The Zinc in quinoa is good for the production of testosterone, the sex hormone that boosts sexual desire, sexual arousal, sex drive and libido in both men and women. Zinc in combination with B vitamins is excellent for sperm count and fertility. Healthy zinc level in the body is same as healthy testosterone level in the body. Healthy testosterone level in the body (male and female) means high sex drive or high libido.

Iron in quinoa is good for the formation of new blood cells. Adequate formation of blood cells aid circulation and nutrients are easily taken to destinations and in this case to the genitals. Red blood cells are good for transporting oxygen to the cells of the body including the tissues of the genitals. Adequate supply of oxygen is dependent on healthy blood platelets and in turn dependent on iron supply to the body blood system.

The B-vitamins in quinoa: Vitamin B6 in quinoa helps the body to produce and secrete testosterone, testosterone is excellent for sex drive. This also helps to maintain general hormonal balance. Zinc in combination with B6 and B9 raises sperm production, sperm count or heavy cum, motility and testosterone production. Low levels of zinc in the body system have been since linked to poor libido in men and women.

Magnesium in quinoa is good for nerve functions, and formation of cell membranes. Magnesium is also essential in the production of sex hormones like androgen, estrogen and neurotransmitters (dopamine and norepinephrine) that regulates libido. Magnesium helps dilate blood vessels. Vaso-dilation improves blood circulation including the supply of blood to the genitals. Better blood flow to the genitals, creates greater arousal for men and women. Adequate blood supply to the genitals is good for sexual desire and sexual arousal.

Add more quinoa to your diet, for sexual health benefits including sex hormone production and balance, sexual desire, sexual arousal, sex drive and libido.

AVOCADOS

Avocados have high-quality Vitamin E content that can boost sexual desire, sexual arousal and intensify orgasm. Vitamin E is popularly known as reproductive vitamin.

Other nutrients in avocado include:

Vitamin B6 – Help the body to produce and secrete testosterone, testosterone is excellent for sex drive.

Potassium – Helps for the proper functioning of the muscles, and is very essential in relaxing the blood vessels – Vasodilation, and encourages healthy blood circulation in the vessels and capillaries. Potassium activates nitric oxide, which relaxes the arteries, reducing the pressure on the arteries and encourages optimal flow and circulation of blood. In so doing, potassium aids in supplying adequate nutrients to the genitals.

Potassium is also very essential for the proper functioning of the thyroid.

Folic acid – Helps to metabolize protein to release energy and stamina. In combination with B vitamins, folic acid is good for fertility. The lack of Vitamin B2, B6 and folic acid have been linked to infertility.

Avocados are good for your libido.

BANANAS

Bananas contain the bromelain enzyme. Bromelain enzyme is known to increase libido, enhance male fertility and reverse erectile dysfunction and impotence in men. Bananas are also good source of Vitamin B6, Vitamin C, manganese, potassium, magnesium and some zinc.

Vitamin B6 in banana helps the body to produce and secrete testosterone - testosterone is excellent for sex drive. This also helps to maintain general hormonal balance.

Potassium regulates the functions of the muscles and is very good for blood circulation thus aiding the supply of blood and nutrients to the genitals. Other nutrients in bananas include B vitamins such as riboflavin. Riboflavin in combination potassium helps the production of testosterone. Potassium is also essential for the proper functioning of the thyroid which is involved in the production sex hormones.

Potassium is very essential in relaxing the blood vessels – Vasodilation, and encourages healthy blood circulation in the vessels and capillaries. Potassium activates nitric oxide, which relaxes the arteries, reducing the pressure on the arteries and encourages optimal flow and circulation of blood. In so doing, potassium aids in supplying adequate nutrients to the genitals.

Manganese in banana is essential for the synthesis of fatty acids, which is necessary for a healthy nervous system. The nervous system is the electrical system of the body.

Magnesium in banana is good for nerve functions, and formation of cell membranes. Magnesium is also essential in the production of sex hormones like androgen, estrogen and neurotransmitters (dopamine and norepinephrine) that regulates libido. Magnesium helps dilate blood vessels. Vaso-dilation improves blood circulation including the supply of blood to the genitals. Better blood flow to the genitals, creates greater arousal for men and women. Adequate blood supply to the genitals is good for sexual desire and sexual arousal.

The Zinc in banana is good for the production of testosterone, the sex hormone that boosts sexual desire, sexual arousal, sex drive and libido in both men and women. Zinc in combination with B vitamins is excellent for sperm count and fertility. Healthy zinc level in the body is same as healthy testosterone level in the body. Healthy testosterone level in the body (male and female) means high sex drive or high libido.

Extra Info: FYI:- Consumption of banana is associated/credited with reduced risk of colorectal cancer, breast cancer and renal carcinoma.

Banana contains the enzyme and amino acid tyrosine which aids (a precursor) the production of dopamine. Banana therefore is friendly to the production of the endorphin, dopamine – a feel-good hormone.

Juice extracted from Banana Corm when mixed with honey to make juice could be good for treating kidney stone and jaundice.

PEANUTS/PEANUT BUTTER

Peanuts are a rich natural source of the amino acid, L-arginine, which is essential for increasing sexual stamina in men and sexual desire, sexual arousal in women. L-arginine relaxes the blood vessels in the penis causing more blood flow to the region, and increasing sexual stamina during sex. Peanuts are also good source of niacin, folate, magnesium, manganese, copper, and vitamin E, phosphorous, zinc, iron, B-vitamins and other monounsaturated fatty acids such as oleic acids.

L-arginine helps to stimulate the release of growth hormone (GH), dopamine and other substances into the body system.

Growth hormones and dopamine help in the production of testosterone which is essential for sexual desire, sexual arousal, sex drive and healthy libido.

L-arginine induces the release of nitric oxide in the body. Nitric acid relaxes the arteries, reducing the pressure on the arteries, reducing blood vessels stiffness and encourages optimal flow and circulation of blood. In so doing, nitric oxide aids the supply of adequate nutrients to the genitals.

L-arginine has been used to treat erectile dysfunction. It helps relax muscles around blood vessels in the penis.

When the blood vessel around the penis dilates, blood flow increases so a man can achieve and maintain an erection.

In this sense, L-arginine therefore aids the function of Nervi eregentis, which is responsible for the erection of the penis.

This is also good for the female libido by aiding blood flow to the genitals. Blood engorgement of the female sex organ is a primer for sexual desire, sexual arousal, sex drive and libido.

Magnesium in peanuts is essential for energy metabolism, proper functioning of the muscle in the body system including vaginal wall muscles and pelvic floor muscles. Magnesium is also good for nerve functions, and formation of cell membranes. Magnesium is also essential in the production of sex hormones like androgen, estrogen and neurotransmitters (dopamine and norepinephrine) that regulates libido. Magnesium helps dilate blood vessels. Vaso-dilation improves blood circulation including the supply of blood to the genitals. Better blood flow to the genitals, creates greater arousal for men and women. Adequate blood supply to the genitals is good for sexual desire and sexual arousal.

Phosphorus is a vital part of all body process as regards growth and maintenance of bones and teeth.

Phosphorous in combination with calcium provides strength to bones. Deficiency of phosphorous may lead to weakness, tooth decay, rickets and other related bone problems.

Testosterone is often and truly associated with the muscle mass of a man. It also plays a role in maintaining the bones, since most body muscles are attached to the bones. Low testosterone is a risk factor of developing osteoporosis – bone disease due to weak bones. The decrease in muscle mass is often associated with decrease in bone density and bone strength. Phosphorous therefore works in indirect support of testosterone and sex drive/libido.

The Zinc in peanuts is good for the production of testosterone, the sex hormone that boosts sexual desire, sexual arousal, sex drive and libido in both men and women. Zinc in combination with B vitamins is excellent for sperm count and fertility. Healthy zinc level in the body is same as healthy testosterone level in the body. Healthy testosterone level in the body (male and female) means high sex drive or high libido.

Manganese in peanuts is essential for the synthesis of fatty acids, which is necessary for a healthy nervous system. The nervous system is the electrical system of the body.

Cooper in peanuts is good for the health of the body's nervous system.

Vitamin E is the sex, reproductive and fertility vitamin.

Iron in peanuts is good for the making of hemoglobin in the red blood cells. Red blood cells are good in taking nutrients and mainly oxygen to the cells and tissues of the body system, including the cells and tissues of the genitals.

Folate in peanuts helps to enhance the reach of orgasm in both male and female, because it aids in the release of histamine. Histamine is excellent in aiding erection, sexual arousal and orgasm in both men and women. Histamine also aids in the release of testosterone, the sex drive hormone. Histamine is released by cell bodies (neurons) called histaminergics which is located at the back of the hypothalamus. Histamine is released as a neurotransmitter in the brain.

Remember the love hormone – Oxytocin? It peaks in the brain and body system during orgasm. Oxytocin is manufactured in the hypothalamus and stored in the thyroid gland. Looks like histamine and oxytocin works very closely.

Does it now make sense to you why people eat banana with peanuts?

See the profile for banana and make the connection.

You see people do certain things without knowing why and as such may be doing the right thing at a thing that is not really opportune.

ALMONDS

Almonds are better eaten raw and without salt for the best result. Nutrients in Almonds include:

Vitamin E – Well known for its function in fertility and reproduction

Essential fatty acids - Fatty acids are essential for the production of male hormones to regulate sex drive.

CELERY

Celery contains androsterone, an odorless hormone and sometimes called pheromone, which is released through male perspiration and turns women on. Celery has high content of Potassium about 8 to 10% of the daily average body daily need.

Potassium is very essential in relaxing the blood vessels – Vasodilation, and encourages healthy blood circulation in the vessels and capillaries. Potassium activates nitric oxide, which relaxes the arteries, reducing the pressure on the arteries and encourages optimal flow and circulation of blood. In so doing, potassium aids in supplying adequate nutrients to the genitals.

Celery also contains some Riboflavin (B2), Folate (B9) and chlorophyll. Riboflavin and folic acid are known fertility aids.

Celery contains high levels of phthalides and coumarins. Phthalin is good in combating high levels of the bad cholesterol (Low density Cholesterol – LDL) in the body system and prevents high blood pressure while providing healthy environment for the production of sex hormone.

OYESTER (Raw)

Oysters contain high in zinc, which raises sperm production (sperm count or heavy cum) and testosterone production. Oysters also contain dopamine boosting nutrients, a hormone known to induce a feel good mood and increase libido. Low levels of zinc in the body system have been since linked to poor libido in men and women. In the male body, zinc is more abundantly situated in the prostate. Zinc in combination with folate Vitamin B9 is excellent for sperm count and fertility. Healthy zinc level in the body is same as healthy testosterone level in the body. Healthy testosterone level in the body (male and female) means high sex drive or high libido.

Oysters contain reasonable levels of Selenium. Selenium assists sperm production and also aid sperm motility. Selenium is most abundantly situated in the seminal ducts and the testes.

PECANS

Pecans are good source of protein and both monounsaturated and polyunsaturated fats including L-arginine.

Pecan is also very rich source of manganese, magnesium, phosphorous, zinc, thiamine, and Iron.

L-arginine in pecan helps to stimulate the release of growth hormone (GH), dopamine and other substances into the body system.

Growth hormones and dopamine help in the production of testosterone which is essential for sexual desire, sexual arousal, sex drive and healthy libido.

L-arginine induces the release of nitric oxide in the body. Nitric acid relaxes the arteries, reducing the pressure on the arteries, reducing blood vessels stiffness and encourages optimal flow and circulation of blood. In so doing, nitric oxide aids the supply of adequate nutrients to the genitals.

L-arginine has been used to treat erectile dysfunction. It helps relax muscles around blood vessels in the penis.

When the blood vessel around the penis dilates, blood flow increases so a man can achieve and maintain an erection.

In this sense, L-arginine therefore aids the function of Nervi eregentis, which is responsible for the erection of the penis.

This is also good for the female libido by aiding blood flow to the genitals. Blood engorgement of the female sex organ is a primer for sexual desire, sexual arousal, sex drive and libido.

Magnesium in pecan is essential for energy metabolism, proper functioning of the muscle in the body system including vaginal wall muscles and pelvic floor muscles. Magnesium is also good for nerve functions, and formation of cell membranes. Magnesium is also essential in the production of sex hormones like androgen, estrogen and neurotransmitters (dopamine and norepinephrine) that regulates libido. Magnesium helps dilate blood vessels. Vaso-dilation improves blood circulation including the supply of blood to the genitals. Better blood flow to the genitals, creates greater arousal for men and women. Adequate blood supply to the genitals is good for sexual desire and sexual arousal.

Zinc in pecan is good for the production of testosterone, the sex hormone that boosts sexual desire, sexual arousal, sex drive and libido in both men and women. Zinc in combination with B vitamins is excellent for sperm count and fertility. Healthy zinc level in the body is same as healthy testosterone level in the body. Healthy testosterone level in the body (male and female) means high sex drive or high libido.

Manganese in pecan is essential for the synthesis of fatty acids, which is necessary for a healthy nervous system. The nervous system is the electrical system of the body.

Vitamin E is the sex, reproductive and fertility vitamin.

Iron in pecan is good for the making of hemoglobin in the red blood cells. Red blood cells are good in taking nutrients and mainly oxygen to the cells and tissues of the body system, including the cells and tissues of the genitals.

Phosphorus is a vital part of all body process as regards growth and maintenance of bones and teeth.

Phosphorous in combination with calcium provides strength to bones. Deficiency of phosphorous may lead to weakness, tooth decay, rickets and other related bone problems.

Testosterone is often and truly associated with the muscle mass of a man. It also plays a role in maintaining the bones, since most body muscles are attached to the bones. Low testosterone is a risk factor of developing osteoporosis – bone disease due to weak bones. The decrease in muscle mass is often associated with decrease in bone density and bone strength. Phosphorous therefore works in indirect support of testosterone and sex drive/libido.

Extra info - FYI:

A diet rich in pecan nuts can lower the risk of gallstone in women.

The antioxidants and phytosterols present in pecans reduce high cholesterol by eliminating the LDL (bad Cholesterol) while preserving the HDL (good cholesterol).

Daily consumption of a handful of pecans may help lower cholesterol (LDL) levels just the same way the marketed cholesterol lowering medication do. It is good to know that most of the so-called cholesterol lowering medications are extracted phytosterols (plant sterols) marketed as cytellin. Daily consumption of pecans may delay age-related muscle nerve degeneration, and muscle wasting or losing.

OATMEAL And Other Whole Grains

Eating oatmeal and whole grains such as wheat help to boost testosterone level in the bloodstream. Testosterones boosts sex drive and intensify orgasm in both men and women. Oats and whole grains contain L-arginine, and other essential fatty acids. L-arginine is an amino acid that enhances the effect of nitric oxide. Nitric acid is a gas molecule that relaxes the arteries, reducing the pressure on the arteries, reducing blood vessels stiffness and encourages optimal flow and circulation of blood. In so doing, nitric oxide aids the supply of adequate nutrients to the genitals. L-arginine has been used to treat erectile dysfunction. It helps relax muscles around blood vessels in the penis. When the blood vessel around the penis dilates, blood flow increases so a man can achieve and maintain an erection. In this sense, L-arginine therefore aids the function of Nervi eregentis. Other whole grains that act exactly like oatmeal includes whole-grain bread, whole wheat bread, brown rice, and barley.

WHEAT GERM

Wheat contains a lot of Vitamin E. Vitamin E is essential for sex and fertility. Vitamin E contains an antioxidant that protects cells from the damages of free-radical. Most important for this topic is that Vitamin E helps the body to synthesize sex hormones, mainly estrogen which is very essential for the body hormonal balance for healthy sex drive and libido. Vitamin E also helps balance estrogen in women's bodies. When a woman's estrogen level is in balance and the woman is in healthy hormonal balance, other hormones including progesterone and testosterone are presumed to be at balance also. And this is good for sex drive and libido. Proper estrogen balance means reduced PMS, anxiety issues, headaches and mood swings and improves sex drive. Wheat germ is also rich in omega-3 fatty acids and other healthy fats.

FATTY FISH

Fatty fishes including salmon, mackerel, sardines, and tuna should contain omega-3 fatty acids with DHA and EPA. DHA and EPA help to raise dopamine levels in the brain. Dopamine helps to produce feel good mood and also help the production of the sex hormone testosterone. Testosterone is essential for sexual desire, and sexual arousal, it is the chief hormone for healthy sex drive and libido. Clinical studies have also demonstrated that omega-3 fatty acids can also reduce symptoms of depression. Depression is not good for sex drive and libido.

Omega 3 fatty acids in fatty fishes contain the amino acid, L-arginine, which stimulates the release of growth hormone (GH) among other substances and is converted into nitric oxide in the body. L-arginine is an amino acid that enhances the effect of nitric oxide. Nitric acid relaxes the arteries, reducing the pressure on the arteries, reducing blood vessels stiffness and encourages optimal flow and circulation of blood. In so doing, nitric oxide aids the supply of adequate nutrients to the genitals. L-arginine has been used to treat erectile dysfunction. It helps relax capillaries around blood vessels in the penis. When the blood vessel around the penis dilates, blood flow increases so a man can achieve and maintain an erection. In this sense, L-arginine therefore aids the function of Nervi eregentis. This is also good for the female libido by aiding blood flow to the genitals. Fatty fishes also help to maintain the levels of HDL – High density cholesterol (good Cholesterol) in the body system, by lowering the levels of the LDL. Fatty fishes contain Monounsaturated and polyunsaturated fats. Cholesterol is essential for the production of the sex hormone in the body.

L-ARGININE

L-arginine is an amino acid found in proteins and fatty acids. Arginine is a nonessential amino acid, meaning it can be manufactured by the human body, and does not necessarily need to be obtained through the diet. However, the biosynthetic pathway of this amino acid does not produce sufficient arginine, and as such some need be consumed through diet. L-arginine helps to stimulate the release of growth hormone (GH), dopamine and other substances into the body system.

Growth hormones and dopamine help in the production of testosterone which is essential for sexual desire, sexual arousal, sex drive and healthy libido.

L-arginine induces the release of nitric oxide in the body. Nitric acid is gas molecule that relaxes the arteries, reducing the pressure on the arteries, reducing blood vessels stiffness and encourages optimal flow and circulation of blood. In so doing, nitric oxide aids the supply of adequate nutrients to the genitals.

L-arginine has been used to treat erectile dysfunction. It helps relax muscles around blood vessels in the penis.

When the blood vessel around the penis dilates, blood flow increases so a man can achieve and maintain an erection.

In this sense, L-arginine therefore aids the function of Nervi eregentis, which is responsible for the erection of the penis.

This is also good for the female libido by aiding blood flow to the genitals. Blood engorgement of the female sex organ is a primer for sexual desire, sexual arousal, sex drive and libido.

The absence of arginine from the diet can lead to a reduced production of spermatozoa and reduced sex drive and libido. It is also necessary for proper nutrition.

Foods (plant sources) that contain L-Arginine include:

- ✓ Granola
- ✓ Peanuts
- ✓ Cashews
- ✓ Walnuts
- ✓ Brazil nuts
- ✓ Cocoanut
- ✓ Pecans
- ✓ Soybeans
- ✓ Chickpeas
- ✓ Oat
- ✓ Wheat germ
- ✓ Buckwheat

Seafood Source Includes: Halibut, lobster, salmon, shrimp, snails, tuna.

Diary Sources Includes: cottage cheese, ricotta, milk, yogurt

Animal Sources: Beef, pork, gelatin, poultry, quail, pheasant

L-arginine is also present as food supplement.

DARK CHOCOLATE

Chocolate is made from the cocoa bean, a natural source of theobromine. Dark chocolate also contains a compound called phenylethylamine (PEA). Phenylethylamine aids the release of endorphins in the body system. Phenylethylamine mimics the brain of a person who is in love. It produces the feeling of being in love. Endorphins are the same chemicals that are triggered by kissing, love making, sex, and increases the feelings of attraction between two people. Dark Chocolate therefore promotes the release of endorphins. Endorphins which mean endogenous morphine is endogenous opioid peptides that mimic the actions of neurotransmitters, and as such functions as neurotransmitters. Endorphins are produced in the pituitary and the hypothalamus during exercise, pain (for comfort or reduction of pain), love, orgasm or when you consume something good or spicy. Endorphins produce analgesia and general feeling of well-being. And this is present in dark chocolate. In addition, chocolate contains an amino acid called tryptophan, which helps produce serotonin. Serotonin is helpful in mood-boosting and inducing relaxation.

Dark chocolate also help to boost nitric oxide output. The nitric oxide output theory is because of the fact that theobromine is used as a vasodilator, which means that it makes blood vessels wider. This means that it is good for blood circulation. Theobromine is a myocardial stimulant as well as a vasodilator.

84

It increases heartbeat, but also dilates blood vessels, causing a reduced blood pressure. In so doing it encourages healthy blood circulation and aids the supply of blood to the genitals, a good feature of healthy sex drive and libido. Get some dark chocolates.

SPINARCH(GREEN-VEGETABLES)

Spinach is a potent source of magnesium, which helps dilate blood vessels. Vaso-dilation improves blood circulation including the supply of blood to the genitals. Better blood flow to the genitals, creates greater arousal for men and women. Adequate blood supply to the genitals is good for sexual desire and sexual arousal. Spinach and other members of the cruciferous vegetable family have been shown to contain indole-3-carbinol. Indole-3-carbinol decreases the level of estrogen in the male body system. This is achieved by indole-3-carbinol adhering to the estrogen nerve end receptors (receptor sites) thus preventing the binding of excess estrogen to the receptors. In so doing it helps to prevent estrogen dominance in both male and female, thus promoting hormonal balance and optimal level of testosterone which is a potent primer of sex drive and libido.

Indole-3-carbinol has been shown to be beneficial in treating lupus.

Indole-3-carbinol induces DNA repair in cells and inhibits the growth of cancer cells.

Broccoli consumption is good for prostate health.

Consumption of broccoli may also cause malodorous flatulence. Cruciferous vegetables can be metabolized to sulforaphane, an anti-cancer compound.

Spinach and other green cruciferous vegetables including:

- ✓ Broccoli
- ✓ Brussels sprouts
- ✓ Kale
- ✓ Cabbage,
- ✓ Swiss chard
- ✓ Bok Choy

They are also good sources of vitamin K, vitamin C, magnesium and folate. Folate (vitamin B9) is a good vitamin for fertility and reproductive health.

Folate may also lower blood levels of a harmful substance called homocysteine. Homocysteine is an amino acid that is very unfriendly to the lining of arteries. It encourages plaque to adhere and accumulate on the walls of arteries, increasing the risk of peripheral arterial disease (PAD).

PUMPKIN SEEDS

Pumpkin seeds contain zinc, vitamin E, Vitamin K, potassium and omega-3 fatty acids. Zinc is well known for aiding the production of testosterone, the sex hormone that boosts sexual desire, sexual arousal, sex drive and libido in both men and women. Pumpkin seeds are also rich in the essential fatty acid omega 3, which acts as a precursor of prostaglandins which is an anti-inflammatory agent. Omega-3 fatty acids have DHA and

EPA hormone-like substances that play a key role in sexual health.

Clinical studies have also demonstrated that omega-3 fatty acids can also reduce symptoms of depression. Depression is not good for sex drive and libido.

Omega 3 fatty acids in pumpkin seeds contain the amino acid L-arginine, which stimulates the release of growth hormone (GH) and dopamine. L-arginine is converted into nitric oxide in the body. L-arginine is an amino acid that enhances the effect nitric oxide. Nitric acid relaxes the arteries, reducing the pressure on the arteries, reducing blood vessels stiffness and encourages optimal flow and circulation of blood. In so doing, nitric oxide aids the supply of adequate nutrients to the genitals. L-arginine has been used to treat erectile dysfunction. It helps relax capillaries around blood vessels in the penis. When the blood vessel around the penis dilates, blood flow increases so a man can achieve and maintain an erection. In this sense, L-arginine therefore aids the function of Nervi eregentis. This is also good for the female libido by aiding blood flow to the genitals. Diet rich in pumpkin seeds will enhance potency, sex drive, libido and fertility.

SPICY CHILI PEPPERS

Spicy Chili Peppers contain capsaicin. Capsaicin produces a burning sensation of in the tissues of the mouth and this triggers the release of endorphins that help to give the body a natural sexual high in preparation for love making and sex. Capsaicin in Chili Pepper stimulates nerve endings, thus raising our pulse and making us sweat. Spicy Chili Peppers therefore induces blood circulation and flow, and sweating all over the body. Increased blood circulation/flow means adequate supply of blood to the genitals which may produce sexual arousal.

GARLIC

The scientific name for Garlic is Allium sativum, and it belongs to the onion genre.

Garlic contains allicin which is an antibiotic and antifungal compound. Allicin is responsible for the hot or stinging/burning sensation in the tissues of the mouth which you feel when you eat raw garlic. However, when cooked, allicin is lost in the boiling or cooking, unlike the chili pepper hot-feel that persists after cooking. Just like in chili pepper, the hot-feel from raw garlic touches the efferent nerves and will encourage/trigger the release of endorphins. Endorphins help to give the body a natural sexual high in preparation for love making and sex.

However, the Allicin in garlic is not responsible for the vasodilation capability of garlic.

The vasodilation ability of garlic is the main factor of its ability to improve sexual desire, sexual arousal, sex drive and libido - aphrodisiac potential.

Vasodilation means that it dilates (make wider) the blood vessel causing greater and adequate circulation/flow of blood in the body system, including greater and adequate blood supply to the genitals, inducing sexual arousal, sex drive and libido.

The increase in blood circulation is achieved by the metabolism of garlic, when the poly-sulfides (diallyl disulfide) in garlic is metabolized in the red blood cells (RBCs) into hydrogen sulfides namely allyl methyl sulfide. This compound diallyl-disufide is responsible for the pungent smell of garlic.

The vaso-dilating action (increase in blood flow) could happen within hours of consuming raw garlic and last for some hours. However the garlic breath may be repulsive to a potential partner.

You can mask the garlic breath temporarily by consuming fresh parsley. Eating fresh parsley is also good for sex drive. Parsley has very high levels of vitamin K. Vitamin K which is very good for blood circulation in the capillaries and general capillary health. Vasodilation is good for sexual arousal. The garlic breath persists because the hydrogen sulfide compound (allyl methyl sulfide) is not digestible in the stomach and passes into the blood and stays in the blood for quite some hours that is why the vasodilation effect of eating raw garlic persists for quite a while, passed into the lungs and the skin, and will be excreted in the urine and sweat.

The claim of garlic in reducing blood pressure and atherosclerosis is based on the vasodilation ability.

Garlic or garlic supplement when taken over time or as part of regular diet with enough protein may increase testosterone levels in the body.

Allicin in Garlic help speed recovery from strep throat, hoarseness, in threating common cold, cough and other minor ailments because of its antibiotic properties.

SOY AND SOY PRODUCTS

Soy binds estrogen receptors, which helps the vagina to remain lubricated and combats symptoms of menopause. Soybeans contain high levels of lignans. Lignans are estrogen-like chemicals which have estrogenic activities in the body system.

Vaginal lubrication is a feature of sexual desire, sexual arousal and sex drive/libido. Soy is also beneficial to prostate health. Soy protein contains chemical compounds called isoflavones, which have similar properties to the hormone estrogen. Soy isoflavones have been cited by clinical studies to increases the production of nitric oxide in the body system. Nitric acid relaxes the arteries, reducing the pressure on the arteries, reducing blood vessels stiffness and encourages optimal flow and circulation of blood. In so doing, soy isoflavones in conjunction with the released nitric oxide aids the supply of adequate nutrients and blood to the genitals. Blood flow to the genitals is an all-time primer of sexual desire, sexual arousal, sex drive and libido.

BLACK BEANS AND OTHER LEGUMES

Black beans have high levels of magnesium, folate, iron, phosphorous, and muscle building protein. Protein increases metabolism by helping to build muscle and stall or slow muscle loss that is a natural part of aging. Black beans, and navy beans are full of muscle-building protein: 18 amino acids (with 8 essential amino acids), 19 kinds of oleic acid, unsaturated fatty acid. The iron in black beans is very good to prevent iron deficiency anemia which ails most women of child-bearing and menstruating age. When women experience heavy menstrual cycle loss lots of iron in the process and needs replenishment. Iron is good for the making of hemoglobin in the red blood cells. Red blood cells are good in taking nutrients and mainly oxygen to the cells and tissues of the body system, including the cells and tissues of the genitals.

Magnesium is essential for energy metabolism, proper functioning of the muscle in the body system including vaginal wall muscles and pelvic floor muscles. Magnesium is also good for nerve functions, and formation of cell membranes. Magnesium is also essential in the production of sex hormones like androgen, estrogen and neurotransmitters (dopamine and norepinephrine) that regulates libido. Magnesium helps dilate blood vessels. Vaso-dilation improves blood circulation including the supply of blood to the genitals. Better blood flow to the genitals, creates greater arousal for men and women.

Adequate blood supply to the genitals is good for sexual desire and sexual arousal.

In general, most legumes contain phytoestrogens that are and have about same molecular structure and physiological activity as estrogen and have estrogen-like activity. The said phytoestrogen in legumes help to maintain the hormonal (estrogen) balance in the woman body system.

Phosphorus is a vital part of all body process as regards growth and maintenance of bones and teeth.

Phosphorous in combination with calcium provides strength to bones. Deficiency of phosphorous may lead to weakness, tooth decay, rickets and other related bone problems.

Testosterone is often and truly associated with the muscle mass of a man. It also plays a role in maintaining the bones, since most body muscles are attached to the bones. Low testosterone is a risk factor of developing osteoporosis – bone disease due to weak bones. The decrease in muscle mass is often associated with decrease in bone density and bone strength. Phosphorous therefore works in indirect support of testosterone and sex drive/libido.

BASIL

Basil increases blood circulation. Improves blood circulation means adequate blood supply to the genital areas and to the genitals. Blood supply and blood engorgement of the genitals induces sexual desire and sexual arousal, which are good features of sex drive and libido and is beneficial in stimulating sex drive and boosting fertility. It is said that basil induces more female sex drive and boost female fertility.

ASPARAGUS

Asparagus is a libido booster, which is high in vitamin E (a great sex vitamin). Asparagus is a good source of vitamin E, which helps men and women produce testosterone, a hormone that stimulates both male and female sex drives. Asparagus also contains folate, and folate helps to enhance the reach of orgasm in both male and female. Asparagus contains folate which aids in the release of histamine. Histamine is excellent in aiding erection and sexual arousal in both men and women. Histamine also aids in the release of testosterone.

Asparagus helps to prevent menstrual cramps and its water retention property helps in PMS - Post menstrual stress. Asparagus is a good source of Rutin. Rutin is good for the proper circulation of the blood in the vessels and blood capillaries, and this quality makes it good for the treatment of varicose vein, crow's feet, dark circle around the eye, reduces high blood pressure and general good of the cardiovascular system. Asparagus contains good amount of Vitamin K which is very good for blood circulation in the capillaries and general capillary health. The blood circulatory function of asparagus aids adequate blood innervation of the genitals. Blood supply to the genitals is good for sexual desire, sexual arousal, erection and general sex drive and libido.

EGGS

Eggs are excellent source of Vitamin B5 and Vitamin B6 which are very essential for the maintenance of hormonal balance in the body system. The two B vitamins are also known stress enemies. It is a well-known fact that eggs are good sources of cholesterol. Cholesterol (especially the LDL – low density cholesterol) is not a friend of health. However, cholesterols are the building blocks of sex hormones including estrogen and testosterone. Testosterone is the basic enhancer of sex drive and libido. Eggs are also known to contain zinc. Zinc is well known for aiding the production of testosterone, the sex hormone that boosts sexual desire, sexual arousal, sex drive and libido in both men and women. Zinc in combination with B vitamins is excellent for sperm count and fertility. Healthy zinc level in the body is same as healthy testosterone level in the body. Healthy testosterone level in the body (male and female) means high sex drive or high libido. Eggs are also good source of vitamin A. Vitamin A is essential for the health of the body's epithelial cells and tissues. The internal lining of the genitals including the vaginal wall linings are made up of epithelial cells and tissues. Some men take raw eggs prior to sexual intercourse, see the connection? Well these foods are not quick fix solutions; you need to incorporate them into your daily menu.

BROWN RICE

Brown Rice? Why not rice you may ask? Well, it is still rice and what makes it different from white rice is not only the brown color it wears. The main difference lies in the nutritional content and health benefits.

Brown rice is rice that is only treated to remove the husk which is the protective outermost layer or covering, and it is ready for consumption. In this way it retains all its natural nutrients including the bran and the germ.

White rice is obtained by processing brown rice to remove the bran and the germ layer and under further polishing to get shiny white rice.

Brown rice is whole grain. It contains Vitamin B6, Niacin, Selenium, Magnesium, Manganese, Zinc, potassium, glutamic acid (an amino acid).

Vitamin B6 in brown rice is essential for the body to produce and secrete testosterone; testosterone is excellent for sex drive and libido. Vitamin B6 aids the absorption of selenium in its dietary form. Vitamin B6 helps both males and females to attain orgasm. Vitamin B6 helps in the general wellbeing of the nervous system.

Vitamin B3 (niacin) is good for metabolism and release of energy from food, thus preventing fatigue. Fatigue is an enemy of libido.

Selenium in brown rice assists sperm production and also aid sperm motility. Selenium is most abundantly situated in the seminal ducts and the testes.

Magnesium in brown rice is essential for energy metabolism, proper functioning of the muscle in the body system including vaginal wall muscles and pelvic floor muscles. Magnesium is also good for nerve functions, and formation of cell membranes. Magnesium is also essential in the production of sex hormones like androgen, estrogen and neurotransmitters (dopamine and norepinephrine) that regulates libido. Magnesium helps dilate blood vessels. Vaso-dilation improves blood circulation including the supply of blood to the genitals. Better blood flow to the genitals, creates greater arousal for men and women. Adequate blood supply to the genitals is good for sexual desire and sexual arousal.

Manganese in brown rice is essential for the synthesis of fatty acids, which is necessary for a healthy nervous system.

The Zinc in brown rice is well known for aiding the production of testosterone, the sex hormone that boosts sexual desire, sexual arousal, sex drive and libido in both men and women. Zinc in combination with B vitamins is excellent for sperm count and fertility. Zinc in combination with selenium is essential for sperm production and sperm motility. Healthy zinc level in the body is same as healthy testosterone level in the body. Healthy testosterone level in the body (male and female) means high sex drive or high libido.

Potassium in brown rice helps for the proper functioning of the muscles, and is very essential in relaxing the blood vessels – Vasodilation, and encourages healthy blood circulation in the vessels and capillaries. Potassium activates nitric oxide, which relaxes the arteries, reducing the pressure on the arteries and encourages optimal flow and circulation of blood. In so doing, potassium aids in supplying adequate nutrients to the genitals. Potassium is also very essential for the proper functioning of the thyroid.

The glutamic acid in brown rice in combination with vitamin B6 aids the production of neurotransmitters, gamma-butyric acid (GABA).

YAM

Yam when consumed with spinach, olive oil and chili pepper could be a potent aphrodisiac. See the profile of:

Olive oil - Vitamin E + Omega-3 fatty acids

Spinach - Spinach is a potent source of magnesium, which helps dilate blood vessels. Vaso-dilation improves blood circulation including the supply of blood to the genitals. Better blood flow to the genitals, creates greater arousal for men and women. Adequate blood supply to the genitals is good for sexual desire and sexual arousal.

Chili Pepper - Spicy Chili Peppers contain capsaicin. Capsaicin produces a burning sensation of in any tissues of the mouth and this triggers the release of endorphins that help to give the body a natural sexual high in preparation for love making and sex.

The yam could be mashed together with spinach and chili pepper, add some olive oil and season to taste just as you prepare mashed potato.

The scientific name for the yam family is Dioscareaceae. Damiana or wild yam grows in Mexico, Central America and West Africa. In West Africa some varieties of the yam are domestic and are called *"Ji Abana"* and another is wild and called *"Ji Nmuo"* in Igbo language (Eastern Nigeria), and yet another popular variety is called *"Ji"*. They are all very potent and occur in different sizes and colors including colors such as yellow, yellowish green, white and reddish-brown. The scientific name for Damiana or wild yam is Turnera diffusa. Wild yam is used in treating impotence. Damiana or wild yam helps to maintain hormonal balance in the body system and also has mildly stimulating properties. Yam contains significant levels of magnesium. It also has high levels of *diosgenin – a steroidal ponins*, which has impact on hormonal pattern and balance.

Wild yam extract may help in the treatment of vaginal dryness and other symptoms of menopause. Asian, oriental, Central American herbalists and naturopathic doctors have recommended wild yam extract for centuries in the treatment of a variety of menstrual and vaginal symptoms. Consuming wild yam and yellow yam have also been said to be very helpful in treating vaginal dryness.

The Steroid Diosgenin, a steroid sapogenin is extracted from yam including the West African yam (ji), mainly from the species of Dioscorea, such as Dioscorea nipponica. Diosgenin is used for the synthesis (commercial) of progesterone, cortisone, and pregnenolone and some other steroids. The manufactured steroids such as progesterone are then used in some contraceptive pills. Unmodified steroids as found in yams are useful phytochemicals that have estrogenic activities in the body system. They act mainly by reducing the amount of cholesterol in the blood stream thereby regulating the synthesis of estrogen and binding of estrogen to the estrogen receptors. This is a good reason for the use of yam in and as phytoestrogen for regulating estrogen levels in the body.

OKRA

Okra is very low in calories and contains good amount of vitamin A, Thiamin, Vitamin B6, vitamin C, folic acid, vitamin B2 riboflavin, calcium, zinc and dietary fiber. Eating okra is much recommended for pregnant woman, because, besides being rich in other nutrients, it is rich in folic acid which is essential for the neural tube formation of the fetus during first 4-12 weeks of gestation period in the mother's womb.

Okra seeds contain protein and amino acids such as tryptophan and cysteine.

Vitamin B6 in Okra – Help the body to produce and secrete testosterone, testosterone is excellent for sex drive

Folic acid – Helps to metabolize protein to release energy and stamina. In combination with other B vitamins, folic acid is good for fertility. The lack of Vitamin B2, B6 and folic acid (B9) have been linked to infertility.

Riboflavin in combination potassium helps the production of testosterone.

Zinc in combination with B vitamins raises sperm production (sperm count or heavy cum) and testosterone production. Low levels of zinc in the body system have been since linked to poor libido in men and women. In the male body, zinc is more abundantly situated in the prostate. Zinc in combination with folate Vitamin B9 is excellent for sperm count and fertility. Healthy zinc level in the body is same as healthy testosterone level in the body. Healthy testosterone level in the body (male and female) means high sex drive or high libido.

Tryptophan helps produce serotonin. Serotonin is helpful in mood-boosting and inducing relaxation.

CRABS AND LOBSTERS

Crab and lobsters are sea foods and they are rich in:

Zinc, Copper, Potassium, Phosphorous, Manganese, Vitamin K, Vitamin A, Vitamin E, Vitamin B12, Iron, Folate Vitamin B9, and Omega-3 fatty acids.

Zinc in combination with folate Vitamin B9 is excellent for sperm count and fertility.

Potassium – Helps for the proper functioning of the muscles, and is very essential in relaxing the blood vessels – Vasodilation, and encourages healthy blood circulation in the vessels and capillaries. Potassium activates nitric oxide, which relaxes the arteries, reducing the pressure on the arteries and encourages optimal flow and circulation of blood. In so doing, potassium aids in supplying adequate nutrients to the genitals.

Manganese is essential for the synthesis of fatty acids, which is necessary for a healthy nervous system.

Vitamin K is very good for blood circulation in the capillaries and general capillary health. The blood circulatory function of vitamin K aids adequate blood innervation of the genitals.

Vitamin E helps the body to synthesize sex hormones, mainly estrogen which is very essential for the body hormonal balance for healthy sex drive and libido.

Omega-3 fatty acids contain DHA and EPA. DHA and EPA help to raise dopamine levels in the brain. Dopamine helps to produce feel good mood and also help the production of the sex hormone testosterone. Testosterone is essential for sexual desire, and sexual arousal, it is the chief hormone for healthy sex drive and libido.

Phosphorus is a vital part of all body process as regards growth and maintenance of bones and teeth.

Phosphorous in combination with calcium provides strength to bones. Deficiency of phosphorous may lead to weakness, tooth decay, rickets and other related bone problems.

Testosterone is often and truly associated with the muscle mass of a man. It also plays a role in maintaining the bones, since most body muscles are attached to the bones. Low testosterone is a risk factor of developing osteoporosis – bone disease due to weak bones. The decrease in muscle mass is often associated with decrease in bone density and bone strength. Phosphorous therefore works in indirect support of testosterone and sex drive/libido.

PRUNES, HAZELNUTS, PEANUTS, KIWI, PLUM, PEAR

All contain reasonable amounts of boron. Boron is a trace mineral/element. Boron increases levels of estrogen in women and testosterone in men. It is used to help regulate sex hormones, especially in women going through menopause, and diminishes the need for Hormone replacement therapy (HRT). Boron regimen in premenopausal, menopausal and postmenopausal women presents fast result in improved sex drive and libido. Symptom of menopause such as hot flashes and depression were quickly eliminated in women undergoing boron regimen. Adequate levels of boron are required for healthy mental function. Boron is good to ward off depression and memory loss. Depression leads to low sex drive/low libido. Boron plays an important role in maintaining trans-membrane functions and in stabilizing the hormone reception. Boron is essential for the metabolism of minerals such as calcium, magnesium and copper. Foods rich in boron are almonds, prunes, avocados and hazelnuts. Other sources of Boron are Kiwi, red grapes, dates, pear, plum, onion, pea nuts butter, lentil, etc.

Boron is good and has shown success in the treatment of arthritis and rheumatoid arthritis. Dietary sources of boron are excellent. However, one can overdose on supplemental boron. Boron could become toxic in high doses. Use with care.

OXYTOCIN

Oxytocin is a hormone and neurotransmitter. Oxytocin hormone works as a transmitter in the human brain, and has been widely used for years for inducing labor, to prevent postpartum or postnatal depression and to induce milk ejection. Clinical studies suggest that the hormone oxytocin can help improve lovers' interactions, which help them to communicate better. In other words, oxytocin improves amorous expression and communication. In addition, Oxytocin can even enhance warmth between strangers.

Oxytocin hinders the release of hormones responsible for stress known as cortisol, and also reduces blood pressures that occur due to anxiety. It makes one feel relaxed, calm, affectionate, generous, trusting and calm. Furthermore, it also improves sociability and reduces the feeling of isolation.

Oxytocin also reduces cravings and dependency, a property that makes it the key to healing addictions of all kinds including hard drugs such as heroin and cocaine.

Touch and hugs prompts the release of oxytocin, leading to feelings of closeness, sexual intimacy, and the release of more oxytocin. Orgasm produces a peak in the hormone about two times the normal level. This accounts for the post-coital calm, relaxation and intimacy and feeling of stronger bond.

Oxytocin in the body system is secreted by the posterior pituitary gland. The pituitary gland stores and releases when need be, oxytocin produced by the hypothalamus.

Oxytocin enhances and intensifies orgasmic experiences. In men, oxytocin helps to establish quick emotional bonding and desire. While in women, quick emotional bonding, desire and multiple orgasms is especially enhanced.

Oxytocin is available and sold as nasal spray called Syntocinon and Pitocin, however, the efficacy of this product as spray is not clearly established. However, producers are saying that intranasal administration of oxytocin causes a substantial increase in trusting behavior and bonding.

Oxytocin can be released by various types of sensory stimulations such as touch and warmth.

PROBABLE INDUCERS OF OXYTOCIN INCLUDE:

MASSAGE

As said earlier touch and hug enhances the release of oxytocin. Using that standard, Oxytocin therefore can be released by various types of sensory stimulation, for example by touch and warmth. Bloodstream levels of oxytocin have been shown to rise during massage. Massage is mainly touch based. It is therefore good therapy for the release of oxytocin.

EXERCISE

Exercise brings the release of endorphins and also wards off depression. Some exercise has been touted to induce labour. By that standard, it is possible that exercise may help to induce the secretion of oxytocin in normal non-pregnant males and females.

Omega-3 fatty acids – (linseeds oil, flax seed, fatty fish, supplement)

Omaega-3 fatty acids and especially from the listed sources contain tryptophan which aids the release of serotonin from the pituitary gland.

Okra

Okra seeds contain tryptophan which aids the release of serotonin from the pituitary gland. Serotonin is a neurotransmitter and is helpful in mood-boosting and inducing relaxation.

Chili Pepper

Capsaicin in chili pepper produces a burning sensation of in any tissues of the mouth and this triggers the release of endorphins that help to give the body a natural sexual high in preparation for love making and sex. Capsaicin in Chili Pepper stimulates nerve endings (efferent nerves), thus raising our pulse and trigger the release of endorphins.

Oxytocin hinders the release of hormones responsible for stress known as cortisol, and also reduces blood pressures that occur due to anxiety. Therefore oxytocin or endorphins may be released in response to provocation caused by chili peppers.

LETTUCE

Lettuce is a rich source of Vitamin K, Vitamin A, Folate – Vitamin B9 and Lactucarium (sometimes called Lettuce Opium). Lactucarium is the milk-like/opiate-like white substance that oozes out from base stem of lettuce when cut. This substance has sedative and analgesic property and as such is sometimes used to induce sleep by eating lettuce. Lactucarium is present in almost all varieties of lettuce but most abundant in Lactuca virosa variety of lettuce. Lactucarium can be collected into a thick solid, and it has proven to have some psychoactive effects or mild hallucination effects

Folate in lettuce helps to enhance the reach of orgasm in both male and female, because it aids in the release of histamine. Histamine is excellent in aiding erection, sexual arousal and orgasm in both men and women. Histamine also aids in the release of testosterone, the sex drive hormone. Histamine is released by cell bodies (neurons) called histaminergics which is located at the back of the hypothalamus. Histamine is released as a neurotransmitter in the brain.

Vitamin K in lettuce is very good for blood circulation in the capillaries and general capillary health. The blood circulatory function of vitamin K in lettuce aids adequate blood innervation of the genitals. Blood supply to the genitals is good for sexual desire, sexual arousal, erection and general sex drive and libido.

KELP/ALGAE/SEAWEED

Kelp or algae extract is derived from seaweed. Kelp, a seaweed is a rich source of iodine, calcium, zinc, magnesium, selenium and iron, Vitamin B9 -folate, Vitamins A and K, and amino acids – L-Lysine.

Iodine was first discovered in 1812 in kelp (seaweed). Iodine in combination with selenium is utilized for the production of thyroid hormones. Thyroid hormone is responsible for the regulation of general metabolism. Selenium assists sperm production and also aid sperm motility. Selenium is most abundantly situated in the seminal ducts and the testes.

Zinc raises sperm production (sperm count or heavy cum) and testosterone production. Low levels of zinc in the body system have been since linked to poor libido in men and women. In the male body, zinc is more abundantly situated in the prostate. Zinc in combination with folate Vitamin B9 is excellent for sperm count and fertility. Healthy zinc level in the body is same as healthy testosterone level in the body. Healthy testosterone level in the body (male and female) means high sex drive or high libido.

Magnesium helps dilate blood vessels. Vaso-dilation improves blood circulation including the supply of blood to the genitals. Better blood flow to the genitals, creates greater arousal for men and women. Adequate blood supply to the genitals is good for sexual desire and sexual arousal.

Magnesium is also essential for energy metabolism, proper functioning of the muscle in the body system including vaginal wall muscles and pelvic floor muscles. Magnesium is also good for nerve functions, and formation of cell membranes. Magnesium is also essential in the production of sex hormones like androgen, estrogen and neurotransmitters (dopamine and norepinephrine) that regulates libido. Dopamine produce feel-good mood that is good for sex drive and high libido.

Iodine deficiency is the major cause of hypothyroidism and goiter, a situation that invariably leads to low sex drive, libido, and in some cases erectile dysfunction (impotence).

Deficiency of thyroid hormones causes chronic fatigue. Fatigue is an enemy of healthy sex drive/libido.

Kelp has a normalizing effect on the thyroid gland. Kelp is also good for the treatment of constipation. Constipation is not good for hormonal balance and sex drive/libido. Kelp is reported to be very beneficial to brain tissue, the membrane surrounding the brain, the sensory nerves, and the spinal cord.

Vitamin A facilitates the efficient absorption of nutrients by strengthening the lining of the digestive tract. The lining of digestive tract is made up of epithelial cells. Vitamin A is essential for the health, maintenance and proper functioning of epithelial cells and tissues. Along with vitamins C and E, it bolsters the immune system. Vitamin A is also necessary for the production of thyroxin, a thyroid hormone, and helps the thyroid to absorb iodine; a key nutrient. Iodine in Kelp maintains a healthy thyroid, thereby significantly reducing one major cause of obesity. Obesity is an enemy of healthy sex drive and libido.

Sources of iodine includes: Kelp, Other seaweed, onion, sushi, etc.

CAVIAR

Eggs harvested from most notably unfertilized sturgeon and salmon. There are red and black caviar. Roe or fish eggs could be harvested from Beluga Sturgeon, Sevruga or Stellate Sturgeon, Dog Salmon, Pink Salmon. Beluga is the largest of sturgeon fishes with the largest caviar.

Caviar contains nutrients such as: selenium, iron, magnesium, calcium and phosphorus, phospholipids and omega-3 fatty acids, omega-6 fatty acids, potassium, vitamin D, vitamin A, vitamin E,

Selenium in caviar helps sperm production and also aid sperm motility. Selenium is most abundantly situated in the seminal ducts and the testes.

Iron in caviar is good for the making of hemoglobin in the red blood cells. Red blood cells are good in taking nutrients and mainly oxygen to the cells and tissues of the body system, including the cells and tissues of the genitals.

Magnesium in caviar is essential for energy metabolism, proper functioning of the muscle in the body system including vaginal wall muscles and pelvic floor muscles. Magnesium is also good for nerve functions, and formation of cell membranes. Magnesium is also essential in the production of sex hormones like androgen, estrogen and neurotransmitters (dopamine and norepinephrine) that regulates libido. Magnesium helps dilate blood vessels. Vaso-dilation improves blood circulation including the supply of blood to the genitals. Better blood flow to the genitals, creates greater arousal for men and women. Adequate blood supply to the genitals is good for sexual desire and sexual arousal.

Potassium in caviar helps for the proper functioning of the muscles, and is very essential in relaxing the blood vessels – Vasodilation, and encourages healthy blood circulation in the vessels and capillaries. Potassium activates nitric oxide, which relaxes the arteries, reducing the pressure on the arteries and encourages optimal flow and circulation of blood. In so doing, potassium aids in supplying adequate nutrients to the genitals.

Potassium is also very essential for the proper functioning of the thyroid.

Omega-3 and omega-6 fatty acids (essential amino acids) contain DHA and EPA. DHA and EPA help to raise dopamine levels in the brain. Dopamine helps to produce feel good mood and also help the production of the sex hormone testosterone. Testosterone is essential for sexual desire, and sexual arousal, it is the chief hormone for healthy sex drive and libido. Clinical studies have also demonstrated that omega-3 fatty acids can also reduce symptoms of depression. Depression is not good for sex drive and libido.

Essential amino acids in caviar contain the amino acid L-arginine, which stimulates the release of growth hormone (GH) among other substances and is converted into nitric oxide in the body. L-arginine is an amino acid that enhances the effect nitric oxide. Nitric acid relaxes the arteries, reducing the pressure on the arteries, reducing blood vessels stiffness and encourages optimal flow and circulation of blood. In so doing, nitric oxide aids the supply of adequate nutrients to the genitals. L-arginine has been used to treat erectile dysfunction. It helps relax capillaries around blood vessels in the penis. When the blood vessel around the penis dilates, blood flow increases so a man can achieve and maintain an erection. In this sense, L-arginine therefore aids the function of Nervi eregentis. This is also good for the female libido by aiding blood flow to and the engorgement of the female the genitalia. Caviar also helps to maintain LDL (Low density cholesterol, Bad Cholesterol) at low levels of and the High density cholesterol (HDL – good cholesterol) at high levels in the bod system, as they contain Monounsaturated and polyunsaturated fats. Cholesterol is essential for the production of the sex hormone in the body.

PINENUTS

Pine nuts contain both monounsaturated and polyunsaturated fatty acids. Pine nuts are also rich sources of zinc, phosphorous, manganese, magnesium, vitamin K, Vitamin E, B-vitamins such as niacin B3 and Thiamine B1.

The L-arginine is present in the unsaturated fatty acids in pine nuts. L-arginine helps to stimulate the release of growth hormone (GH), dopamine and other substances into the body system.

Growth hormones and dopamine help in the production of testosterone which is essential for sexual desire, sexual arousal, sex drive and healthy libido.

L-arginine induces the release of nitric oxide in the body. Nitric acid relaxes the arteries, reducing the pressure on the arteries, reducing blood vessels stiffness and encourages optimal flow and circulation of blood. In so doing, nitric oxide aids the supply of adequate nutrients to the genitals.

L-arginine has been used to treat erectile dysfunction. It helps relax muscles around blood vessels in the penis.

When the blood vessel around the penis dilates, blood flow increases so a man can achieve and maintain an erection.

In this sense, L-arginine therefore aids the function of Nervi eregentis, which is responsible for the erection of the penis.

This is also good for the female libido by aiding blood flow to the genitals. Blood engorgement of the female sex organ is a primer for sexual desire, sexual arousal, sex drive and libido.

Magnesium in pine nuts is essential for energy metabolism, proper functioning of the muscle in the body system including vaginal wall muscles and pelvic floor muscles. Magnesium is also good for nerve functions, and formation of cell membranes. Magnesium is also essential in the production of sex hormones like androgen, estrogen and neurotransmitters (dopamine and norepinephrine) that regulates libido. Magnesium helps dilate blood vessels. Vaso-dilation improves blood circulation including the supply of blood to the genitals. Better blood flow to the genitals, creates greater arousal for men and women. Adequate blood supply to the genitals is good for sexual desire and sexual arousal.

The Zinc in pine nuts is good for the production of testosterone, the sex hormone that boosts sexual desire, sexual arousal, sex drive and libido in both men and women. Zinc in combination with B vitamins is excellent for sperm count and fertility. Healthy zinc level in the body is same as healthy testosterone level in the body. Healthy testosterone level in the body (male and female) means high sex drive or high libido.

Manganese in pine nuts is essential for the synthesis of fatty acids, which is necessary for a healthy nervous system. The nervous system is the electrical system of the body.

Vitamin E contains an antioxidant that protects cells from the damages of free-radical. Most important for this topic is that Vitamin E helps the body to synthesize sex hormones, mainly estrogen which is very essential for the body hormonal balance for healthy sex drive and libido. Vitamin E also helps balance estrogen in women's bodies. When a woman's estrogen level is in balance and the woman is in healthy hormonal balance, other hormones including progesterone and testosterone are presumed to be at balance also. And this is good for sex drive and libido. Good estrogen balance means reduced PMS, anxiety issues, headaches and mood swings. Without these problems, her sex drive is bound to improve.

Vitamin K in pine nuts is very good for blood circulation in the capillaries and general capillary health. The blood circulatory function of vitamin K aids adequate blood innervation of the genitals. Adequate supply of blood to the genitals is a known primer for sexual desire, sexual arousal, sex drive and libido.

B vitamins in combination with Zinc are excellent for sperm count and fertility.

Pine nuts or pine nuts cookies devoured with cup of dark espresso elevates sex drive.

Extra Info: FYI:- Pine-nut oil may suppress appetite. It does so by releasing endogenous cholecystokinin (CCK - a satiety gut hormone)

MUSTARD SEED

Mustard seeds from mustard plant. Mustard seeds are excellent source of magnesium, zinc, phosphorous, calcium, vitamin B1, vitamin B2, vitamin B6, Iron, vitamin E and folate. Mustard seeds also contain good amount of monounsaturated and polyunsaturated fatty acids including Omega-3 fatty acids.

Mustard seeds are used to make a mustard condiment, mustard paste, mustard spice, and mustard powder. They range in colour from yellow to dark brown.

Magnesium in mustard seeds helps dilate blood vessels. Vaso-dilation improves blood circulation including the supply of blood to the genitals. Better blood flow to the genitals, creates greater arousal for men and women. Adequate blood supply to the genitals is good for sexual desire and sexual arousal. Magnesium is also important for bone, muscles and connective tissue health.

The Zinc in mustard seeds is well known for aiding the production of testosterone, the sex hormone that boosts sexual desire, sexual arousal, sex drive and libido in both men and women. Zinc in combination B vitamins is excellent for sperm count and fertility. Healthy zinc level in the body is same as healthy testosterone level in the body. Healthy testosterone level in the body (male and female) means high sex drive or high libido.

Vitamin B6 in mustard seeds help the body to produce and secrete testosterone, testosterone is excellent for sex drive. This also helps to maintain general hormonal balance.

Omega-3 and omega-6 fatty acids (essential amino acids) contain DHA and EPA. DHA and EPA help to raise dopamine levels in the brain. Dopamine helps to produce feel good mood and also help the production of the sex hormone testosterone. Testosterone is essential for sexual desire, and sexual arousal, it is the chief hormone for healthy sex drive and libido. Clinical studies have also demonstrated that omega-3 fatty acids can also reduce symptoms of depression. Depression is not good for sex drive and libido.

Essential amino acids in caviar contain the amino acid L-arginine, which stimulates the release of growth hormone (GH) among other substances and is converted into nitric oxide in the body. L-arginine is an amino acid that enhances the effect of nitric oxide. Nitric acid relaxes the arteries, reducing the pressure on the arteries, reducing blood vessels stiffness and encourages optimal flow and circulation of blood. In so doing, nitric oxide aids the supply of adequate nutrients to the genitals. L-arginine has been used to treat erectile dysfunction. It helps relax capillaries around blood vessels in the penis. When the blood vessel around the penis dilates, blood flow increases so a man can achieve and maintain an erection. In this sense, L-arginine therefore aids the function of Nervi eregentis. This is also good for the female libido by aiding blood flow to the genitals.

Phosphorus is a vital part of all body process as regards growth and maintenance of bones and teeth.

Phosphorous in combination with calcium provides strength to bones. Deficiency of phosphorous may lead to weakness, tooth decay, rickets and other related bone problems.

Testosterone is often and truly associated with the muscle mass of a man. It also plays a role in maintaining the bones, since most body muscles are attached to the bones. Low testosterone is a risk factor of developing osteoporosis – bone disease due to weak bones. The decrease in muscle mass is often associated with decrease in bone density and bone strength. Phosphorous therefore works in indirect support of testosterone and sex drive/libido.

FRUITS

WATERMELON

Watermelon contains beta-carotene, lycopene and citrulline. Citrulline is converted into L-arginine in the body via nitric oxide synthase. L-arginine induces the release of nitric oxide in the body system. Nitric oxide is a gas molecule that help smooth muscle in arterioles dilate and relax (vasodilation), thereby increasing blood flow. Vasodilation encourages healthy blood circulation in the vessels and capillaries reducing the pressure on the arteries and encourages optimal flow and circulation of blood. In so doing aids in engorging and supplying adequate nutrients to the genitals. Blood supply to the genitals is an all-time primer of sexual desire, sexual arousal, sex drive and libido. It is said that there is more citrulline in the rinds (whitish part) of watermelon. Citrulline and L-arginine is suitable for the treatment of erectile dysfunction.

Lycopene in watermelon is good for prostate health, and prevents prostate cancer.

NUTMEG

Nutmeg is the roughly egg-shaped seed of the Nutmeg tree. The nutmeg tree is of the genus Myristica.

The common or fragrant nutmeg tree, *Myristica fragrans*, is a native of the Banda Islands of Indonesia. It is also grown in Penang Island of Malaysia, the Caribbean and Grenada.

The active ingredients in the seed of the nutmeg are: Elemicin, and Myristicin

Large dose of raw and freshly ground nutmeg produces psychoactive, hallucinations and euphoric effects on users.

Elemicin is a phenylpropene (a natural organic anticholinergenic compound) and causes an anticholinergic-like effect on a person. As an anticholinergenic, elemicin blocks the action of the neurotransmitter acetylcholine in the both the Central Nervous System (CNS – Brain + Spinal cord) and the Peripheral Nervous system (blood vessels and nerves besides brain and spinal cord) from binding to its receptor nerves cells/fibers. The nerve fibers of the parasympathetic system are responsible for the involuntary movements of smooth muscles present in body such as: Urinary tract/bladder, pelvic floor muscles, genital muscles, lungs, etc.

During intercourse and orgasm, the smooth muscles of the genitals contracts involuntarily for orgasm to happen. The anticholinergenic effect of elemicin prolongs and helps you to control the contraction of the PC/genital muscles.

Nutmeg's elemicin is a neuromuscular blocker and could be useful in treating urinary incontinence.

Anticholinergenics are divided into three categories to represent their targets in the central and/or peripheral nervous system:

antimuscarinic agents, ganglionic blockers, and neuromuscular blockers.

Other examples of anticholinergenics include: atropine and dicycloverine

Myristicin belongs to the class of monoamine oxidase inhibitors (MAOIs). Monoamine oxidase inhibitors are a class of antidepressant drugs, used in the treatment of atypical/unusual/light depression. This is what provides the euphoria from nutmeg.

Myristicin is responsible for the euphoria and the hallucination.

PINEAPPLE

Rich in bromelain, magnesium, calcium, potassium, fiber, and vitamin C. Bromelain is considered an effective anti-inflammatory agent. Anti-inflammatory refers to the property of a substance or treatment that reduces inflammation. Anti-inflammatory drugs make up about half of analgesics (pain relievers), remedying pain by reducing inflammation. Anti-inflammatory agents induce analgesic feeling, which is an ok-feeling or all-is-good kind of feeling. Ok-feeling is a typical feeling of love, sexual desire and sexual arousal.

Magnesium in pineapple helps dilate blood vessels. Vaso-dilation improves blood circulation including the supply of blood to the genitals. Better blood flow to the genitals, creates greater arousal for men and women. Adequate blood supply to the genitals is good for sexual desire and sexual arousal.

Magnesium is also important for bone, muscles and connective tissue health.

Potassium in pineapple helps for the proper functioning of the muscles, and is very essential in relaxing the blood vessels – Vasodilation, and encourages healthy blood circulation in the vessels and capillaries. Potassium activates nitric oxide, which relaxes the arteries, reducing the pressure on the arteries and encourages optimal flow and circulation of blood. In so doing, potassium aids in supplying adequate nutrients to the genitals. Potassium is also very essential for the proper functioning of the thyroid. Bromelain has been found quite effective acting as a non-steroidal anti-inflammatory (NSAIDs) in relieving pain that comes from osteoarthritis and rheumatoid arthritis. Bromelain has long been used to treat connective tissue disorders such as scleroderma, tendonitis, and bursitis.

BLUEBERRIES, RASPBERRIES AND STRAWBERRIES

Strawberries contain vitamin C, vitamin K, manganese, folate, potassium, riboflavin, vitamin B5, vitamin B6, copper, magnesium and anthocyanin.

Blueberries contain vitamin A, niacin, iron and Vitamin C, vitamin B6, vitamin C, vitamin K and essential mineral such as manganese. In addition, Blueberries contain anthocyanins, proanthocyanins, resveratrol, flavonols and tanins.

Proanthocyanidins are condensed tannins. Proanthocyanidins are vasoactive polyphenols: meaning that they act on blood vessels. Proanthocyanidins suppress production of a protein endothelin-1 that constricts blood vessels. By working against vaso-constriction, proanthocyanidins are vasodilators. Proanthocyanidins induces and optimize the production of nitric oxide in the artery walls relaxing them and reduced pressure thus allowing greater and adequate blood flow.

The action of nitric oxide activation and subsequent vasodilation that encourages healthy blood circulation in the vessels and capillaries and which relaxes the arteries, reducing the pressure on the arteries and encourages optimal flow and circulation of blood and adequate nutrients to the genitals, forms the main bases of berries being good for sex drive. This is so true understanding that blood flow to the penis and engorgement of the female genitals are primers of sexual desire, sexual arousal and sex drive/libido.

Proanthocyanidins also play a role in the stabilization of collagen and maintenance of elastin. Collagen and elastin are structural proteins that are very important for the health of connective tissue that support organs, joints, blood vessels, lungs and muscles. The penis is made up of muscular fibers. The vaginal canal is lined with vaginal muscles.

Vitamin K in berries is very good for blood circulation in the capillaries and general capillary health. The blood circulatory function of vitamin K in berries aids adequate blood innervation of the genitals. Blood supply to the genitals is good for sexual desire, sexual arousal, erection and general sex drive and libido.

GOJI BERRY

Goji Berry, otherwise called Wolfberry is from the specie Lycium Barbarum of the family Solanaceae. Other plants in the Solanaceae family includes: tobacco, chili pepper, eggplant, deadly nightshade, potato and tomato.

Goji Berry is a native of mainly Asia and Southeastern Europe. Most of the commercially available Goji berries are from north-central and western china. In the said regions of china, they are grown in plantations.

Goji Berries are rich sources of the following:

Atropine which is also found in most of the Solanaceae family of plants is an anti-cholenergenic.

Phytochemicals such as five unsaturated fatty acids including essential fatty acids such as Alpha-linoleic acid (polyunsaturated - omega-3 fatty acid) and gamma-linoleic acid (polyunsaturated - omega-6 fatty acid), and other 18 amino acid.

High levels of **minerals** such as Potassium, high levels of Zinc, very high level of Iron and very high levels of selenium

Very high levels of **Vitamins** including Vitamin C and Vitamin B2. Other nutrients in Goji berries are Beta-carotene, lutien, Zeaxanthin, lycopene, cryptoxanthin and xanthophyll. Beta-sitosterol and phyosterols are also present in Goji berries. Polysaccharides make up about a third of the pulp weight of a Goji berry fruit.

Potassium in Goji Berries helps for the proper functioning of the muscles, and is very essential in relaxing the blood vessels – Vasodilation, and encourages healthy blood circulation in the vessels and capillaries. Potassium activates nitric oxide, which relaxes the arteries, reducing the pressure on the arteries and encourages optimal flow and circulation of blood. In so doing, potassium aids in supplying adequate nutrients to the genitals. Potassium is also very essential for the proper functioning of the thyroid. The Zinc in Goji Berries is good for the production of testosterone, the sex hormone that boosts sexual desire, sexual arousal, sex drive and libido in both men and women. Zinc in combination with B vitamins is excellent for sperm count and fertility. Healthy zinc level in the body is same as healthy testosterone level in the body. Healthy testosterone level in the body (male and female) means high sex drive or high libido. Low levels of zinc in the body system have been since linked to poor libido in men and women. Iron in Goji Berries is good for the formation of new blood cells. Adequate formation of blood cells aid circulation and nutrients are easily taken to destinations and in this case to the genitals. Red blood cells are good for transporting oxygen to the cells of the body including the tissues of the genitals. Adequate supply of oxygen is dependent on healthy blood platelets and in turn dependent on iron supply to the body blood system. Selenium in goji berries assists sperm production and also aid sperm motility. Selenium is most abundantly situated in the seminal ducts and the testes.

Lycopene in goji berries is good for prostate health.

FIGS

Figs are excellent source of minerals like calcium, copper, potassium, manganese, iron, selenium and zinc. Potassium is very good to control high blood pressure and low intake of potassium can lead to hypertension.

Manganese in figs is essential for the synthesis of fatty acids, which is necessary for a healthy nervous system.

The Zinc in figs is well known for aiding the production of testosterone, the sex hormone that boosts sexual desire, sexual arousal, sex drive and libido in both men and women. Zinc in combination with vitamin C and also B vitamins are excellent for sperm count and fertility. Healthy zinc level in the body is same as healthy testosterone level in the body. Healthy testosterone level in the body (male and female) means high sex drive or high libido.

Potassium in figs helps for the proper functioning of the muscles, and is very essential in relaxing the blood vessels – Vasodilation, and encourages healthy blood circulation in the vessels and capillaries. Potassium activates nitric oxide, which relaxes the arteries, reducing the pressure on the arteries and encourages optimal flow and circulation of blood. In so doing, potassium aids in supplying adequate nutrients to the genitals. Potassium is also very essential for the proper functioning of the thyroid.

Selenium in figs is utilized for the production of thyroid hormones. Thyroid hormone is responsible for the regulation of general metabolism. Selenium assists sperm production and also aid sperm motility. Selenium is most abundantly situated in the seminal ducts and the testes.

DATES

Though dates contain other nutrients and minerals, but 80% of the nutritional content is made up of sugar (fructose). Other nutrients include: Potassium, Magnesium and manganese and B vitamins. Dates is not a quick fix fruit or aphrodisiac; however, the high sugar content may provide immediate energy, warding off fatigue, but not sex drive, sexual desire or arousal.

BL

CHAPTER 8

HERBS AND ROOTS TO IMPROVE LIBIDO

MANJAKANI OR OAK GALL (for Women)

The word Manjakani is Malay language for Oak Gall. Manjakani or oak gall is popularly consumed in Malaysia, Indonesia and South East Asia by women after birth and generally by nursing mothers. It is believed and proven that the tonic herbal drink has positive effect on tone and tighten vaginal muscles after childbirth. Oak Galls is produced by the activities of stinging wasps on the leaves of the oak tree. Oak Gall is a round hard ball which is formed from chemical reaction arising from secretions by various insects most especially the stinging wasp as they penetrate the leaves of Oak tree leaves to lay eggs and other activities.

Oak Gall is very rich in calcium, iron, vitamins A and C, tannins, tannic acid, gallic acid, fiber, protein and carbohydrates. Oak gall has astringent properties that help in toning, tightening and firming the vaginal wall muscles. It restores vaginal wall elasticity and tone. In addition, assists in reducing vaginal discharge called leucorrhoea which causes bad vaginal odor and also eliminates vaginal itching. Its antiseptic properties are very effective in fighting vaginal yeast, bacterial and fungal infection.

CURCUMA COMOSA (for Women)

Curcuma comosa is a species of flowering plant of the Ginger family. The herb is a native of Asia. It is most popularly cultivated in Thailand, in the Northern provinces of Thailand, particularly in Petchaboon, and the Northeastern Province, Loei. Clinical research shows that curcuma comosa increases the thickness of epithelial cells lining the vaginal canal.

The vagina canal is made up of squamous and stratified epithelial muscles. It is also reported to have aided the repair of vaginal wall prolapse. Vaginal wall prolapse as we discussed in the earlier chapters is a sign and symptom of Loose Vagina. Curcuma Comosa therefore is entirely good for tightening vaginal and love muscles. They have been reported to help in relieving vaginal dryness, bad odor, promote circulation to the female genitals, tone saggy muscles and have estrogenic effect. They are said to help make skin glow.

Curcuma Comosa pills may be available in Herbal stores.

BLACKCOHOSH (for Women)

Black cohosh is a perennial plant that is a member of the buttercup family. Other common names for blackcohosh are:

black snakeroot, bugwort, etc. The scientific name is for black cohosh is cimicifuga racemosa.

Content/Ingredients in Blackcohosh: Phytochemicals such as beta-carotene, phytosterols, salicylic acid and tannin, calcium, iron, magnesium, phosphorous and B5 vitamin, vitamin A, actaeine, cimicifungin, estrogenic substances, glycosides, isoferulic acid, isoflavones, oleic acid, palmitic acid, racemosin, formononetin, triterpenes, and triterpene saponins. Blackcohosh simulates the effects of estrogen.

It may help strengthen the muscles in the pelvic floor, relaxes uterine muscle spasms, thus its suggested use for the treatment of urinary incontinence. It is also used for the treatment of vaginal dryness and hot flashes in menopausal women.

In some cases, it has been used to treat depression, anxiety and arthritis.

Black cohosh supplements are derived from the roots and underground stems (called rhizomes) of the black cohosh plant. There are suggestions about the potency of the leaves.

GINSENG

Consuming Ginseng has been said to have positive effects on female hormonal levels. This helps in toning and healthful maintenance of vaginal wall muscles. Consuming ginseng greatly reduces vaginal dryness and painful sexual intercourse.

The active ingredient in Ginseng is gensinosides. Ginseng is known to possess phytoestrogens.

These effects of ginseng as sex drive enhancer may not be due to changes in hormone secretion.

The libido enhancing ability of ginseng is mostly due to it active ingredient (ginsenoside) effect on the central nervous system and gonadal tissues.

In males, ginsenosides can facilitate penile erection.

Ginseng has been demonstrated to have a stimulating effect on the pituitary gland to increase the secretion of gonadotropins.

Side effects may include: high blood pressure or low blood pressure. It is not advisable to mix ginseng with antidepressants.

DAMIANA OR WILD YAM (EXTRACT)

The scientific name for the general yam family is Dioscareaceae. The scientific name for Damiana or wild yam is Turnera diffusa. Damiana or wild yam grows in Mexico, Central America and West Africa. In West Africa some varieties of the yam are domestic and is called *"Ji Abana"* and another is wild and called *"Ji Nmuo"* in Igbo language (Eastern Nigeria), and yet another domestic variety is called *"Ji"*. They are all very potent and occur in different sizes and colors including colors such as yellow, yellowish green, white and reddish-brown. Wild yam is used in treating impotence. Damiana or wild yam helps to maintain hormonal balance in the body system and also has mildly stimulating properties. Yam contains significant levels of magnesium. It also has high levels of *diosgenin – a steroidal ponins*, which has impact on hormonal pattern and balance.

Wild yam extract may help in the treatment of vaginal dryness and other symptoms of menopause. Asian, oriental, Central American herbalists and naturopathic doctors have recommended wild yam extract for centuries in the treatment of a variety of menstrual and vaginal symptoms. Consuming wild yam and yellow yam have also been said to be very helpful in treating vaginal dryness.

The Steroid Diosgenin, a steroid sapogenin is extracted from yam including the West African yam (ji), mainly from the species of Dioscorea, such as Dioscorea nipponica. Diosgenin is used for the synthesis (commercial) of progesterone, cortisone, and pregnenolone and some other steroids. The manufactured steroids such as progesterone are then used in some contraceptive pills. Unmodified steroids as found in yams are useful phytochemicals that have estrogenic activities in the body system. They act mainly by reducing the amount of cholesterol in the blood stream thereby regulating the synthesis of estrogen and binding of estrogen to the estrogen receptors. This is a good reason for the use of yam in and as phytoestrogen for regulating estrogen levels in the body. Consuming yam in its natural form therefore is good.

DONG QUAI (Women's)

Angelica sinensis, commonly known as Dong quai is herb from the Apiaceae family of the plant kingdom. The plant is a native of china. Dong quai is not good for pregnant women because it may increase the risk of miscarriage. It is best used by premenstrual and menopausal women. Dong Quai is an aromatic herb and an oriental herb that grows abundantly in China, Korea, and Japan. Herbalists use Dong Quai in the treatment of a variety of gynecological complications including vaginal dryness, painful sexual intercourse, and regulation of menstrual as well as menopausal problems. Dong Quai contains vitamin E, B12, and A. It is also very rich in tannins and tannic acid. Other phytochemicals in the herb includes coumarins, phytosterols, polysaccharides, ferulate, and flavonoids. It also has analgesic, sedative and anti-inflammatory properties. It may also reduce blood pressure and fatigue.

EPINEDIUM SAGITTATUM – HORNY GOAT WEED (men's)

The horny goat weed herb is mainly found in Asia and the Mediterranean. The Chinese call it Yin Yang Huo, and it means "sexy goat plant" There are various species and varieties of the plant. However, all the specie contains the active ingredient (icariin) to different degrees. Horny goat weed is known to have other sexual health and general health benefits. Icariin works by increasing levels of nitric oxide nitric oxide, which relaxes the arteries, reducing the pressure on the arteries and encourages optimal flow and circulation of blood to the genitals, encouraging lasting erection. Icariin is a phytoestrogen, and works by blocking the activity of a particular enzyme phosphodiesterase-5 (PDE-5) in the body, with similar effect of some prescription drugs that treat erectile dysfunction such as Viagra. Healthy blood supply to the genitals means supply of nutrients to the cells, tissues and muscles of the genitals including vaginal wall muscles. Furthermore, some flavonoids in some species of horny goat weed have flavonoid with potent and specific estrogen receptor (ER) bioactivity. Studies in laboratory animals show that horny goat weed may influence levels of neurotransmitters such as norepinephrine, serotonin, and dopamine and reduce cortisol levels.

The herb/leaves of horny goat weed may be used frequently; however, the supplement is better used on an intermittent basis. The herbal supplement may be available from drug and herbal stores.

TRIBULUS TERRESTRIS

Tribulus terrestris is mainly found in China and South Africa. In china, it is a traditional herb. It's used to enhance sexual function, increase muscle mass, urinary incontinence, and improve sperm motility, improve sperm count/volume, sex drive, sexual desire, sexual arousal and libido. Some mixtures of different compounds (phytochemicals) found in the fruits, stems and roots of the plant - tribulus terrestris provide its medicinal properties. It's said that such phytochemicals present in tribulus terrestris may encourage increase in the body levels of hormones such as testosterone and dehydroepiandrosterone, or DHEA. Testosterone helps to maintain estrogen balance in the body system, DHEA is converted to estrogen in body and maintains estrogen balance which is essential to reduces vaginal dryness, and curing atrophic vaginitis – proud symptoms of loose vagina.

Good testosterone level in the body improves the time the body muscles needs to recover from any health lapse, and enhances protein synthesis using the body's constituent amino acids. Normal testosterone level also promotes positive estrogen balance. The combination of these actions all help to strengthen and increase the body muscle mass, including vaginal wall muscle and most importantly the sex drive, sexual desire, sexual arousal and libido of both men and women. The only side effects that may be experienced include upset stomach, which can be helped/reduced/eliminated if the herb/supplement is taken with food. The herbal supplement may be available from drug and herbal stores.

HYPOTHETICAL SIDE EFFECT OF TRIBULUS

Caution need be exercised here by **pregnant women and breast-feeding mothers**. Considering that, as explained herein, tribulus terrestris increases testosterone level, it then means that the possibility of side effects may include anger and rage, lowering of the female voice, increased body or facial hair, increase in the size of or an enlarged prostate (already troubled prostate) or the worsening of hormone-related cancer such as breast or prostate cancer.

OTHER FOODS WITH ESTROGEN AND ESTROGEN-LIKE PHYTOCHEMICALS

LIQOURICE (women)

Liquorice is the root of the plant Glycyrrhiza glabra. It is a legume, and the sweet taste is driven from the active ingredient/compound glycyrrhizin (a natural sweetener) and the flavor comes from the compound anethole. It is called Athimathuram in Tamil. In Sanskrit, it is called Yashtimadhu and in Northern India it is called Mulethi. Liquorice flavor is found in a range of liquorice candies reinforced by anise seed oil, tarragon oil or fennel oil because they have similar flavor. The stick and root can be chewed and are available in sweet shops and some herbal shops. Liquorice root induces the production of estrogen, which is essential for sexual functioning. A good level of the hormone estrogen in the woman body system is essential to maintain vaginal health

The active ingredient in liquorice (glycyrrhezenic acid) affects the body's endocrine system. The effect on the endocrine system is because of the isoflavones (Phytoestrogen) content of the gycyrrhezenic acid. The effect reduces the blood level of testosterone, and in so doing help in maintaining hormonal balance mainly beneficial to women.

Consuming liquorice candy in excess may be toxic to the liver, the cardiovascular system and may produce hypertension and edema swelling from accumulation of fluid under the skin).

MACA ROOT

The scientific name for Maca Root is Lepidium Meyenii. It is native to South America and particularly to the Andes and the Inca natives of Peru, Bolivia. It is grown for its fleshy hypocotyl and the taproot. The tap root is used as a medicinal herb and as root vegetable just like carrot.

Phytochemicals present in the Maca root and hypocotyl includes: Uridine, malic, benzoyl, glucosinalates, glucotropaeolin and m-methoxyglucotropaeolin.

The dried roots of Maca contain as much amino acids and fatty acids as in any popular cereal and whole grains. Fatty acids present in Maca are: linolenic acid, palmitric acid, oleic acids and other 19 amino acids.

Mineral content of Maca are Calcium, potassium, Selenium, magnesium, iron, iodine, copper, manganese and zinc.

A chemical in Maca called p-methoxybenzyl isothiocyanate has been touted as responsible among other chemicals for the sex drive/libido qualities of Maca.

Another chemical contained in methanol extract from Maca called methyltetrahydro-carboline-3-carboxylic acid is reported to have effect and acts on the central nervous system.

Maca has also been shown to improve sperm production, sperm motility, and semen volume. Maca help to reduce enlarged prostate.

Iodine in Maca in combination with selenium is utilized for the production of thyroid hormones. Thyroid hormone is responsible for the regulation of general metabolism. Selenium assists sperm production and also aid sperm motility. Selenium is most abundantly situated in the seminal ducts and the testes.

Potassium in Maca helps for the proper functioning of the muscles, and is very essential in relaxing the blood vessels – Vasodilation, and encourages healthy blood circulation in the vessels and capillaries. Potassium activates nitric oxide, which relaxes the arteries, reducing the pressure on the arteries and encourages optimal flow and circulation of blood. In so doing, potassium in Maca aids in supplying adequate nutrients to the genitals. Adequate blood supply to the genitals is good for sexual desire, sexual arousal, sex drive and libido.

Potassium is also very essential for the proper functioning of the thyroid. Potassium is also good for blood circulation, and adequate blood circulation aids sex drive and libido. Potassium helps to control hypertension.

Manganese in Maca is essential for the synthesis of fatty acids, which is necessary for a healthy nervous system. The nervous system is the electrical system of the body.

Magnesium in Maca is good for nerve functions, and formation of cell membranes. Magnesium is also essential in the production of sex hormones like androgen, estrogen and neurotransmitters (dopamine and norepinephrine) that regulates libido. Magnesium helps dilate blood vessels. Vaso-dilation improves blood circulation including the supply of blood to the genitals. Better blood flow to the genitals, creates greater arousal for men and women. Adequate blood supply to the genitals is good for sexual desire and sexual arousal.

The Zinc in Maca is good for the production of testosterone, the sex hormone that boosts sexual desire, sexual arousal, sex drive and libido in both men and women. Zinc in combination with B vitamins is excellent for sperm count and fertility. Healthy zinc level in the body is same as healthy testosterone level in the body. Healthy testosterone level in the body (male and female) means high sex drive or high libido.

HESPERIDIN

Hesperidin is a citrus bioflavonoid. Contents of Hesperin include the flavonoid - flavonne glycoside (glucoside), the flavonne hesperitin, and deschloride rutinose.

Hesperin is very predominant in lemons and peppers. Hesperin is most abundant and concentrated in the rinds and peel of oranges, peppers, lemons and tangerine. Orange juice with pulp has more flavonoids than orange juice without pulp. The combination of vitamin C, rutin and hesperin as found in the said sources is an excellent combination for the health and rejuvenation of epithelial and connective tissues and cells as found in the vaginal wall and the pelvic floor.

Hesperidin and a flavone glycoside diosmin are used to treat and support the health of veins, venous insufficiency and hemorrhoids. Hesperidin is said to be helpful in maintaining capillary health, thus improving circulation and supply of nutrients to epithelial cells and tissues. Hesperidin may also have anti-inflammatory effects.

Because of its assistance in maintaining capillary health, it is said to be very useful in treating varicose veins and bruising. Hesperidin aids blood circulation by relaxing and dilating blood vessels. Vaso-dilation improves blood circulation including the supply of blood to the genitals. Better blood flow to the genitals, creates greater arousal for men and women. Adequate blood supply to the genitals is good for sexual desire and sexual arousal and libido.

Hesperidin in combination with Vitamin C helps to maintain the health of genital muscles especially the collagen and elastic linings of the vaginal canal.

MUIRA PUAMA

The scientific name for muira pauma is Ptychopetalum and it is from the Olacaceae family of the plant kingdom. It is a native of

Brazil, and grows in the Amazon forest. All parts of the plant including the bark, leaves and roots are used for medicinal purposes by the natives in the Rio Negro region of Amazonia, Brazil. Phytochemicals present in Muira puama includes polyunsaturated amino acids such as Omega-3 fatty acid and omega-6 fatty acids. Metabolites from the polyunsaturated fatty acids include L-lysine and L-alanine as we have explained in the previous chapters and pages. L-lysine is excellent for elastin production and L-alanine is good for nitric oxide production in the body system. Both are excellent for sex drive and libido.

Other phytochemicals are phytosterols, coumarin, lupeol (anti-inflammatory agent also present in mango) and muirapuamine – an alkaloid, the active ingredient named after the plant.

The sterols in muira puama are responsible for regulating cholesterol level of the blood thus helping in the maintenance of the hormonal balance of the body system. Remember cholesterol is needed by the body for the production of sex hormones. The alkaloid muira puamine has been said to be responsible for the aphrodisiacs properties of muira puama. Muira puama is available from herbal stores.

SAW PALMETTO: Saw Palmetto is also called Serenoa repens, and it is the only plant specie classified under the genus Serenoa and belongs to the palm family. In some circles, it is known as Sabal serrulatum. The generic name is in honor of the American Botanist Sereno Watson.

Saw palmetto is a palm that reaches a height of about 4.5 maximum (6.2ft). It is mainly found in Southeastern United States including Florida. The palm may live up to 700 years.

The fruits of Saw Palmetto are very rich in fatty acids, Phytosterols, and minerals found in the fruits include high levels of Zinc, Manganese and Magnesium. Fatty acids in Saw palmetto are essential for the production of male hormones to regulate sex drive. Fatty acids such as Omega-3 and Omega-6 fatty acids in Saw palmetto are essential for sex drive and sexual arousal. Omega-3 fatty acids contain DHA and EPA. DHA and EPA help to raise dopamine levels in the brain. Dopamine helps to produce feel good mood and also help the production of the sex hormone testosterone. Testosterone is essential for sexual desire, and sexual arousal, it is the chief hormone for healthy sex drive and libido. Clinical studies have also demonstrated that omega-3 fatty acids can also reduce symptoms of depression. Depression is not good for sex drive and libido.

Omega 3 fatty acids in fatty fishes contain the amino acid L-arginine, which stimulates the release of growth hormone (GH) among other substances and is converted into nitric oxide in the body. L-arginine is an amino acid that enhances the effect of nitric oxide. Nitric oxide relaxes the arteries, reducing the pressure on the arteries, reducing blood vessels stiffness and encourages optimal flow and circulation of blood. In so doing, nitric oxide aids the supply of adequate nutrients to the genitals. L-arginine has been used to treat erectile dysfunction. It helps relax capillaries around blood vessels in the penis. When the blood vessel around the penis dilates, blood flow increases so a man can achieve and maintain an erection. In this sense, L-arginine therefore aids the function of Nervi erigentis. This is also good for the female libido by aiding blood flow to the genitals. The phytosterols in Saw Palmetto help maintain the levels of HDL – High density cholesterol in the body system, by reducing the levels of the LDL – Low density cholesterol. Cholesterol is essential for the production of the sex hormones in the body. Manganese in saw palmetto is essential for the synthesis of fatty acids, which is necessary for a healthy nervous system. The nervous system is the electrical system of the body.

The nervous system regulates the production and secretion of hormones. High level of Zinc in Saw palmetto is good for the production of testosterone, the sex hormone that boosts sexual desire, sexual arousal, sex drive and libido in both men and women. Zinc in combination with B vitamins is excellent for sperm count (semen volume) and fertility. Healthy zinc level in the body is same as healthy testosterone level in the body. Healthy testosterone level in the body (male and female) means high sex drive or high libido. The very high level of Zinc in Saw Palmetto is the main contributor for its use in the treatment of Baldness. Saw palmetto has been shown to help improve the proper functioning of the thyroid gland and thus in maintaining the production of thyroid hormones. Saw palmetto is good for prostate health and particularly prostate hyperplasia. High content of Zinc in saw palmetto is good for sex drive and libido.

Other uses of saw palmetto includes: in respiratory ailment and disorders, prostate cancer, coughs, urinary infections and skin disease such as acne, polycystic ovarian syndrome and hyperandrogen. Herbal supplement of saw palmetto is readily available from herbal and drug stores.

WHITETORN/BLACKTHORN/NATIVE OLIVE

Other names are Mayflower, Prickly pine, Spiny bursaria, Sweet bursaria.

The scientific name for this plant is Bursaria spinosa. It is from the Pittosporaceae family of the plant kingdom. The plant is commonly found in Southern, Western and Northern Australia. It is used in making the drug aesculin. Phytochemicals present in Whitethorn includes Bioflavonoids and Proanthocyanidins.

The leaves, fruits (berries), flower and sometimes the root of Whitethorn have been used to improve sex drive, sexual desire and sexual arousal in women particularly. It has been employed in the treatment of reproductive disorder in both women and men. Proanthocyanidins are condensed tannins. Proanthocyanidins are vasoactive polyphenols: meaning that they act on blood vessels. Proanthocyanidins suppress production of a protein endothelin 1 that constricts blood vessels. By working against vaso-constriction, proanthocyanidins are vasodilators. Proanthocyanidins induces and optimize the production of nitric oxide in the artery walls relaxing them and reduced pressure thus allowing greater and adequate blood flow.

The action of nitric oxide activation and subsequent vasodilation that encourages healthy blood circulation in the vessels and capillaries and which relaxes the arteries, reducing the pressure on the arteries and encourages optimal flow and circulation of blood and adequate nutrients to the genitals, forms the main bases of berries being good for sex drive. This is so true understanding that blood flow to the penis and engorgement of the female genitals are primers of sexual desire, sexual arousal and sex drive/libido.

Proanthocyanidins also play a role in the stabilization of collagen and maintenance of elastin. Collagen and elastin are structural proteins that are very important for the health of connective tissue that support organs, joints, blood vessels, and muscle. The penis is made up of muscular fibers. The active ingredients in Whitethorn have been shown to help in the repair and rejuvenation of epithelial and connective tissues and cells. The vaginal canal is lined with epithelial cells and tissues.

Vitamin K in Whitethorn berries is very good for blood circulation in the capillaries and general capillary health. The blood circulatory function of vitamin K in Whitethorn berries aid adequate blood innervation of the genitals. Blood supply to the genitals is good for sexual desire, sexual arousal, erection and general sex drive and libido.

Bioflavonoids in Whitethorn are helpful in the treatment and support the health of veins, venous insufficiency and hemorrhoids. Whitethorn is said to be helpful maintaining capillary health, thus improving circulation and supply of nutrients to epithelial cells and tissues. Whitethorn may also have anti-inflammatory effects.

Because of its assistance in maintaining capillary health, Whitethorn is said to be very useful in treating varicose veins and bruising. Whitethorn aids blood circulation by relaxing and dilating blood vessels. Vaso-dilation improves blood circulation including the supply of blood to the genitals. Better blood flow to the genitals, creates greater arousal for men and women. Adequate blood supply to the genitals is good for sexual desire and sexual arousal and libido. Whitethorn supplements are available over the counter in most drug stores and herbal shops.

MACUNA PRURIENS

Mucuna Prureins are plants found in Asia, and contains interestingly high levels of isoflavones, Lignans and L-dopa. Other bioactive ingredients in Macuna Pruriens are glutathione, lecithin, venolic acid and gallic acid. Isoflavones are estrogen-like chemicals which have estrogenic activities in the body system. Soy isoflavones have been cited by clinical studies to increases the production of nitric oxide in the body system Nitric acid relaxes the arteries, reducing the pressure on the arteries, reducing blood vessels stiffness and encourages optimal flow and circulation of blood. In so doing, Macuna pruriens isoflavones in conjunction with the released nitric oxide aids the supply of adequate nutrients and blood to the genitals. Blood flow to the genitals is an all-time primer of sexual desire, sexual arousal, sex drive and libido. Macuna pruriens also have effect on the endocrine system and this is because of the isoflavones content. The effect helps in maintaining hormonal balance mainly beneficial to women. Macuna pruriens have been touted to help in strengthening immune system and improving mental clarity.

ASHWAGANDHA

Ashwagandha belongs to the nightshade family without inheriting the vast poisons present in some of the family members. The scientific name of Ashwagandha is Withania somnifera, from the Solanaceae (nightshade) family of the plant kingdom. It is also called India Ginseng or Winter Cherry. It is easy to find out from the Latin name somnifera that the plant may be sleep-inducing. The long brown and tuber-like roots are mainly employed for medicinal uses. The fruits have milk-like coagulating properties. The active ingredients/compound found in this plant are alkaloids, steroidal lactones, atropine, and cuscohygrine. Other active compounds mainly found in the leaves include withanolides, called withaferin A. Active ingredients in Ashwagandha help to maintain hormonal balance, increase testosterone production, cure nervous disorders, enhance stamina and improve vitality. Ashwagandha have been shown to boost sperm count (semen volume), restores erectile function and boosts libido. Ashwagandha may induce abortion and as such is not good for pregnant women.

The compound Withaferin A is helpful in treating colon cancer where it was shown to be anti-metastatic in action. Other medicinal uses includes in treating tumors and tubercular glands. It may also stimulate the thyroid gland. Atropine in Ashwagandha is anticholinergenics and may help to prolong stamina.

RHODIOLA ROSEA

Rhodiola Rosea is also called Golden Root, Roseroot, and Aaron's rod. The plant grows mainly in very cold regions such as Arctic region, Mountains of Central Asia, and mountainous regions of Europe. It belongs to the Crassulaceae family of the plant kingdom. The Chinese name for Rhodiola Rosea is Hóng jǐng tiān. It is mainly used and may be very effective for improving mood and alleviating depression. It is a good-mood herb: - it betters mood and improves sex drive. It has also been shown through clinical research to improve physical strength, anti-fatigue and mental alertness and performance. Its help in physical performance and anti-fatigue means it can improve and sustain sexual stamina and libido. An active ingredient found in Rhodiola Rosea called Rosiridin was shown to inhibit monoamine oxidases (MAO) and this is one reason it has been touted to be good in improving depression and senile dementia.

Other active compounds found in Rhodiola Rosea include Rosavin, Rosarin, Rosin, Rhodioloside and tyrosol, with Rhodioloside and Tyrosol being the most active of the compounds. However, all of the compounds are shown to be phytophenols. Other constituent active ingredients and phytochemicals in Rhodiola rosea are Proanthocyanidins, quercetin, gallic acid and kaempferol. Proanthocyanidins are condensed tannins. Proanthocyanidins are vasoactive polyphenols: meaning that they act on blood vessels. Proanthocyanidins suppress production of a protein endothelin-1 that constricts blood vessels. By working against vaso-constriction, proanthocyanidins are vasodilators. Proanthocyanidins induces and optimize the production of nitric oxide in the artery walls relaxing them and reduced pressure thus allowing greater and adequate blood flow.

The action of nitric oxide activation and subsequent vasodilation that encourages healthy blood circulation in the vessels and capillaries and which relaxes the arteries, reducing the pressure on the arteries and encourages optimal flow and circulation of blood and adequate nutrients to the genitals, forms the main bases of berries being good for sex drive. This is so true understanding that blood flow to the penis and engorgement of the female genitals are primers of sexual desire, sexual arousal and sex drive/libido. Proanthocyanidins also play a role in the stabilization of collagen and maintenance of elastin. Collagen and elastin are structural proteins that are very important for the health of connective tissue that support organs, joints, blood vessels, and muscle. The penis is made up of muscular fibers. The vaginal canal is lined with vaginal muscles. It has also been shown to intensify orgasm in both males and females. They also aid in improving vaginal dryness in premenstrual and menstrual women. The herb and its extract (dried rhizomes) are available from herbal stores and some drug stores.

KAVA

Kava has been said to reduce stress, calm nerves, ward-off depression and improve sex drive and libido. This herb is available from herbal stores, and drug stores everywhere. In Canada and France Kava it is illegal.

GINKGO BILOBA

Ginkgo Biloba is very popular for its ability to improve blood circulation and memory in both men and women. The ingredients in ginkgo biloba help to release nitric oxide in the body system. Nitric oxide helps to open the potassium channel, which causes the blood vessels to relax – vasodilation, and this aids the proper blood circulation and blood supply to the genitals. Adequate blood supply to the genitals aids sexual arousal, sexual desire, sex drive, and libido. This herb is available from herbal stores and drug stores.

CATUABA BARK EXTRACT

Found mainly in South America, Brazil. This plant extract have been touted to help in alleviating lots of health problems including boosting sex drive and libido in both males and females. Other uses of catuaba extract are in:

- ✓ Boosting immune system health
- ✓ Kidney function arthritis
- ✓ Hypertension
- ✓ Obesity
- ✓ Urinary tract healing
- ✓ Priming Brain function

The extract is available in herbal stores and drug stores.

CHAPTER 9

VITAMINS-SUPPLEMENTS-MINERALS
FOR SEX DRIVE AND LIBIDO

Vitamins provide substances that human body may not be producing due to hormonal imbalance, nutritional deficiencies and or because they are essential vitamins. Essential vitamins are those vitamins that the body system does not produce on their own, an example is vitamin C.

VITAMIN E

Vitamin E has been said to aid the production of sex hormones including estrogen and testosterone.

Vitamin E oil sometimes called the sex vitamin is helpful for rejuvenating dry vaginal tissues when taken orally and when used as a topical application. You can get vitamin E from your diet; however, dietary vitamin E may not provide a large enough quantity to supply your body with what you need to overcome low sex drive, dead libido and vaginal dryness. In this light, you may want to take an oral and topical vitamin E oil supplement to aid in relieving your vaginal dryness, vaginal tightness, sexual desire, sexual arousal and libido.

Taking doses of vitamin E, say 400 to 800 IU daily, helps a woman's body produce estriol (building blocks of estrogen) and progesterone to maintain estrogen balance.

Vitamin E is also important for women going through the perimenopause. In general, perimenopause usually start between ages 45 and 49. Almost all symptoms of sex drive and vaginal health in this phase of a woman's life is caused by wild fluctuation in estrogen levels.

Vitamin E helps the body conserve the building blocks of estrogen, estriol, and the progesterone it needs for hormonal balance. Vitamin E aids the supply of nutrients and oxygen to the sex organs by encouraging circulation and supply of blood to the sex organ. Vitamin E also helps to protect the ova from damage. Vitamin E in combination with zinc are good for the body to attain proper functioning of the sex organs including the penile muscles, vagina, vulva, pelvic floor and vaginal wall muscles.

TOPICAL APPLICATION OF VITAMIN E OIL

The topical application of vitamin E oil is mainly for lubrication. Some women use the oil from Vitamin E capsules to replicate vaginal lubrication. Applying Vitamin E oil on a daily basis rehydrates the vaginal tissues. The walls of the vaginal canal incorporate the moisture from vitamin E oil back into its natural processes. Remember the vaginal wall oozes out moisture into the canal during arousal and intercourse. Vitamin E can be used episodically as a lubricant before intercourse.

The use of all natural vitamin E oil is far better and healthier to use in lubricating the vaginal canal and walls than the over-the-counter lubricants. This is because the over-the-counter vaginal lubricants contain drying chemicals or scents.

Use vitamin E oil instead of vaginal lubricants. Vitamin E oil is high in nutrients that nourish the vaginal wall and vaginal muscles. As the vaginal walls absorb the nutrients in vitamin E oil, it heals and alleviates the problems associated with perimenopause, menopause, atrophic vaginitis, vaginal dryness and loose vagina – all are serious culprits of low sex drive and libido. Insert a 400 IU or 800UI vitamin E gel cap into the vagina at bedtime for relief of dryness. As the gel capsule dissolves the vitamin E oil coats delicate vaginal tissues. You may also insert another capsule of vitamin E oil into the vagina as you set off for work. Vitamin E oil is available at health food stores and in most drug stores. Far from the oil of the vitamin E capsule, the capsule itself is mainly made of Gelatin. Gelatin is hydrolyzed collagen and elastin. The vaginal muscles are lined/made-up of collagen and elastin. Elastin is responsible for the folds and coils of the vaginal walls inside the vaginal canal, which is responsible for the elasticity of the vagina. Elastin is also responsible for penile erection (stretching) and recoil. The gelatin dissolves and some may be absorbed and incorporated into the vaginal wall. Elastin and Collagen are both structural proteins and are together responsible for vaginal elasticity and tightness/firmness.

VITAMIN A

Vitamin A maintains the health of the epithelial tissues which line all the external and internal surfaces of the body tissues and organs, including the linings of the vaginal wall and the uterus in women. Vaginal wall consist of stratified squamous epithelial muscles.

Generally, sex hormones including estrogen have DNA receptor sites, and vitamin A is in the family that is friendly to the receptors.

Vitamin A helps in the regulation of the synthesis of the sex hormone, progesterone, which in turn helps in balancing the levels of estrogen and testosterone. Vitamin A has a direct activity towards the regulation of sexual growth, development, and reproduction by turning and switching on genes in response to sex hormone triggers. Vitamin A can also increase hormonal (progesterone) development. Progesterone is associated with improved sexual urge and the power to remain active for a longer time.

BETACAROTENE

Beta-carotene capsules/supplement may also be used in place of Vitamin A. Beta-carotene is converted to vitamin A in the body system and one can never overdose on beta-carotene, nor can the body reach any toxic level of beta-carotene. The conversion of beta-carotene to vitamin A is only done as and when the body needs it. Do not use Beta-carotene and Vitamin A at the same time. It is one or the other, and not together. Carrot is very rich in beta-carotene.

ELASTIN

Elastin or otherwise called tropoelastin is a structural protein responsible for elasticity (stretching and recoil) found mainly in connective tissues such as vaginal wall, the penis, skin, blood vessels (chiefly the aorta), joints, ligaments, cartilages. Elastin allows tissue to resume or return to their original shape/size after stretching or contracting. In this case, it helps the vagina to return to its original size after stretches such as in child-birth, insertion of large objects, and loosening. In the human body, elastin is biochemically coded by the gene known as the ELN. Elastin is made up of randomly coiled fibers of about 830 essential amino acids that are cross-linked into a durable form, and lysine is chiefly responsible for the cross-linkage. The two types of links found in elastin are: desmosine link and isodesmosine link.

Remember the ridges or folds of the vaginal wall? Elastin is responsible for the ridges (coils or folds).

Elastin is also found in the bladder and the lungs (expands when full of urine or air respectively and contracts when emptied).

Deficiency of elastin causes:

General loss of elasticity such as in blood vessels, Loose vagina, Loose bladder (incontinence)

Emphysema (shortness of breath) as in the lungs, caused by alpha-1-antitrypsin deficiency

Marfan's Syndrome

Elastin therefore aids in the health of the blood vessels, as such it is very essential to adequate and proper blood circulation and supply. Proper blood circulation and supply is a primer to erection, sexual desire, sexual arousal, sex drive and libido.

Food Sources of Elastin includes:

Plant sources – Beans, lentils, soy, legumes, pea, amaranth, maize or corn /cornmeal for containing lysine, proline, glycine, alanine, and valine

Animal sources – Bovine, Chicken, Poultry, Pork, non-fat milk, beef, eggs, parmesan cheese

Sea food Sources – fatty fishes, sardine, salmon, caviar, catfish

Gelatin (hydrolyzed collagen)

SUPPLEMENT Forms

Elastin, Lysine, Alanine, Proline, Valine, Glycine, Allysine

COLLAGEN: Collagen like elastin is commonly found in penile tissues, vaginal muscles, connective tissues such as ligaments, blood vessels, skin, bones, eye(cornea)and gut in the form of elongated fibril (strands of fibrillin -glycoproteins). Collagen is created in the body cells called fibroblast. In muscle tissue, it serves as a major component of the endomysium. The endomysium is a layer that covers/en-sheaths the muscle fiber made-up of mostly reticular fibers. There are 28 types of known collagen including:

Type I Collagen - commonly found in the Skin, organs, tendon, vascular ligature, and bone

Type II Collagen – commonly found in the cartilage

Type III Collagen – commonly found in reticular fibers alongside type 1

Type IV Collagen – commonly found in cell membrane base

Type V Collagen – commonly found on cell surfaces, hair, hair follicular base and placenta

Over 90% of the collagen in the body, however, is of type one.

Stress (cortisol) causes the degradation of skin collagen to amino acids.

Type I and Type III collagen are mainly used and imparted during reconstructive surgery, as artificial substitutes.

Why surgery when you can take the substance as supplement and avoid the risks associated with surgery.

SUPPLEMENT Forms

Type I Collagen and Type II Collagen are supplementary collagen for vaginal muscle health, lubrication and tightening. It is also essential for penile stretching and recoil.

However, collagen is a protein and proteins must be metabolized (broken down) into constituents amino acids before absorption, amino acids supplements may offer quicker absorption.

Amino Acid Supplements include: lysine, proline, glycine, alanine, and valine

FOOD SOURCES of Collagen/Amino Acids

Plant sources – Beans, lentils, soy, legumes, pea, amaranth, maize or corn /cornmeal for containing lysine, proline, glycine, alanine, and valine

Animal sources – Bovine, Chicken, Poultry, Pork, non-fat milk, beef, eggs, parmesan cheese

Sea food Sources – fatty fishes, sardine, salmon, caviar, catfish

Gelatin (hydrolyzed collagen)

VITAMIN C

Vitamin C is involved in the synthesis of sex hormones such as androgen, estrogen and progesterone. Vitamin C helps to increase libido and also highly effective in increasing fertility. Vitamin C is essential for the production of collagen and elastin, both forms part of the support to the vaginal attachment to the pelvic floor. Collagen and elastin also forms part of the penis muscular fibers and responsible for penile stretching and recoil. Elastin is the structural protein responsible for the elasticity of the vagina, the vaginal wall and vaginal canal.

VITAMIN D

Vitamin D is an essential part of the endocrine system. Vitamin D helps to regulate several of the adrenal hormones, growth of cells, and production of enzymes. DHEA is produced by the adrenal glands. DHEA or Dehydroepiandrosterone is a steroid hormone produced by the body to create both male and female hormones. DHEA is secreted naturally in the body by the adrenal glands. DHEA and estrogen hormone levels in the body tends to peak in the twenties and decline as people get older. DHEA is converted in the body to both the female hormone, estrogen and the male hormone testosterone.

VITAMIN B6

Vitamin B6 is necessary for metabolism of protein, fat and amino acids, hormonal function (estrogen and testosterone), and the production of red blood cells, niacin, and neurotransmitters (serotonin, norepinephrine, dopamine, GABA –gama-aminobutyric acid). GABA is directly responsible for the regulation of muscle tone including smooth muscles such as vaginal and pc muscles. Vitamin B6 is essential for the general good of the nervous system.

It is very important for keeping stress away.

Vitamin B6 is directly involved in synthesis and secretion of dopamine in the brain; dopamine gives a feel good mood. Feel-good mood is love mood and sex drive friendly.

Vitamin B6 is essential for conversion of selenium in its dietary state (selenomethionine) into an absorbable form by the body.

Vitamin B6 helps in controlling elevated prolactin and in so doing functions as a libido enhancer.

Vitamin B6 helps to balance the levels of progesterone and estrogen. Ingesting Vitamin B6 regularly, helps a woman reach orgasm and sometimes increases sexual stamina of both men and women.

159

VITAMIN B12 + VITAMIN B9

Vitamin B12 may help in improving vaginal dryness by regulating and improving the function of adrenal gland. In regulating the adrenal functions, the B vitamins help to regulate the production of DHEA which is converted to estrogen and is essential to the hormonal balance of the body and to vaginal health, vaginal muscle health, alleviate vaginal dryness and restore vaginal elasticity. Once vaginal elasticity is restored, curing loose vagina and making it tight again is just few Kegels away. Intake of Vitamin B12 in combination with Vitamin B9 (folic acid), may help the body system to function properly. Vitamin B12 is essential to the proper and optimal function of the body system. Vitamin B9 helps to enhance the reach of orgasm in both male and female, because it aids in the release of histamine. Histamine is excellent in aiding erection, sexual arousal and orgasm in both men and women. Histamine also aids in the release of testosterone, the sex drive hormone. Histamine is released by cell bodies (neurons) called histaminergics which is located at the back of the hypothalamus. Histamine is released as a neurotransmitter in the brain. In addition, vitamin B9 also lower blood levels of a harmful substance called homocysteine. Homocysteine is an amino acid that is very unfriendly to the lining of arteries. It encourages plaque to adhere and accumulate on the walls of arteries, increasing the risk of peripheral arterial disease (PAD). Vitamin

B9 is good for general fertility and reproductive health. In pregnant women, vitamin B9 aids the development of neural tubes and the placental links in the first 4 – 12 weeks of gestation. The B vitamins are water soluble and as such are not stored in the body quite unlike the fat soluble vitamins. This means that though the body has a recommended daily value, reaching a toxic level of the B vitamins in the body is not possible, as they could not be stored in the body.

VITAMIN K

Vitamin K is very good for blood circulation in the capillaries and general capillary health. The blood circulatory function of vitamin K aids adequate blood innervation of the genitals. Blood supply to the genitals is good for sexual desire, sexual arousal, erection and general sex drive and libido.

ARGININE OR L-ARGININE

Arginine is an amino acid, also referred to as L-arginine.

It is a very popular amino acid and supplements for sexual dysfunction for both men and women.

Arginine helps stimulates the body to release growth hormone among other substances and is converted into nitric oxide in the body. Nitric oxide is a compound that helps in the health of blood vessels, improving the flow of adequate blood through the arteries and to the sexual organs, including vaginal wall muscles, PC/love muscles. Adequate blood supply to the vaginal wall muscles means good supply of nutrients to the cells and tissues of the vaginal wall muscles. L-Arginine can be taken in herbal pill form. However, many women interviewed report that they achieved the best results by applying a cream directly where it counts. Food rich in L-Arginine includes granola, oatmeal, peanuts, cashews, walnuts, dairy, soybeans, chickpea, seeds and nuts.

L-LYSINE

L-lysine, is an essential amino acid. The human body cannot produce or synthesize lysine. Lysine restores and or promotes the production of arginine in the body system. Lysine helps restore arginine to its normal levels. L-arginine promotes circulation and relaxes blood vessels. L-arginine is essential for the body production of nitric oxide. Nitric oxide helps to open the potassium channel, which causes the blood vessels to relax – vasodilation, and this aids the proper blood circulation and blood supply to the genitals. Adequate blood supply to the genitals aids sexual arousal, sexual desire, sex drive, and libido.

The body system produces its own L-arginine. However, L-lysine aids the arginine to reach its adequate and or optimum level in the body system.

DHEA

DHEA or Dehydroepiandrosterone is a steroid substance produced by the body to create both male and female hormones. DHEA itself is neither a hormone nor a vitamin; however, it is a precursor, aid, primer and or regulator of sex hormones. DHEA is secreted naturally in the body by the adrenal glands. DHEA and estrogen hormone levels in the body tends to peak in the twenties and decline as people get older. DHEA is converted in the body to both the female hormone, estrogen and the male hormone testosterone. Levels of DHEA decline naturally with age and this can lead to decreased estrogen levels and subsequently atrophic vaginitis, vaginal dryness, vaginal itching, decreased sex drive, decreased libido.

DHEA is available over the counter in most drug stores in USA. However, it is good to remember that hormones are precision substances in that at any point, hormones require the proper balance to work effectively. And when you overdose on them, the resulting imbalance may cause health problems rather than improve them. You are therefore advised to consult an experienced professional before employing hormonal replacement therapy and make sure you have the correct dosage and are in good health. DHEA is neither a hormone nor a vitamin, however, it plays a vital role in hormonal production, regulation and balance. Intermittent (off-on) use of this precursor may be safe.

MINERALS FOR SEX DRIVE AND LIBIDO

MAGNESIUM

Magnesium is essential for energy metabolism, proper functioning of the muscle in the body system including vaginal wall muscles, pelvic floor muscles and penile muscles. Magnesium is also good for nerve functions, and formation of cell membranes. Magnesium is also essential in the production of sex hormones like androgen, estrogen and neurotransmitters (dopamine and norepinephrine) that regulates libido.

Deficiency of magnesium in the body may lead to muscle weakness, irregular heartbeat, muscle spasms or twitches. Magnesium is good for energy metabolism and protein synthesis. Magnesium helps dilate blood vessels and as such helps in proper blood circulation to the genitals including the vaginal, vulva, vaginal wall and the penis. Better blood flow to the genitals, creates greater arousal for men and women.

Magnesium-rich foods include artichokes, bananas, dried figs, prune juice, yogurt, spinach and potatoes, leafy green vegetables, seaweed or green algae, avocados, nuts, beans, raw chocolate, and grains such as brown rice and millet.

Magnesium supplements are available over the counter from the drug stores.

SELENIUM

Selenium is vital to ensure the production of healthy ova & sperms. It acts as a coenzyme to calcium and magnesium.

Selenium assists sperm production and also aid sperm motility. Selenium is most abundantly situated in the seminal ducts and the testes.

Foods with high selenium content include Brazil nuts, tuna, oysters, celery, orange rinds and wheat flour.

Vitamin B6 is essential for conversion of selenium in its dietary state (selenomethionine) into an absorbable form by the body.

Selenium supplement is available over the counter in drug stores.

BORON

Boron can influence the production and estrogen metabolism in the body system. While boron supplement works well for some women, it may worsen menopausal symptoms in some other women. Boron is a trace mineral/element, which means its body daily need is small. Boron increases levels of estrogen in women and testosterone in men. It is used to help regulate sex hormones, especially in women going through menopause, and diminishes the need for hormone replacement therapy (HRT). Boron regimen in premenopausal, menopausal and postmenopausal women presents fast result in improved sex drive, libido and vaginal lubrication. Symptom of menopause such as hot flashes and depression were quickly eliminated in women undergoing boron regimen. Adequate levels of boron are required for healthy mental function. Boron is good to ward off depression and memory loss. Depression leads to low sex drive/low libido, and associated dryness. Boron plays an important role in maintaining trans-membrane functions and in stabilizing the hormone reception. Boron is essential for the metabolism of minerals such as calcium, magnesium and copper. Foods rich in boron are almonds, prunes, avocados and hazelnuts. Other sources of Boron are Kiwi, red grapes, dates, pear, plum, onion, pea nuts, peanut butter, lentil, leafy vegetables, and beans etc.

Boron is good and has shown success in the treatment of arthritis and rheumatoid arthritis. Dietary sources of boron are excellent.

Boron is also present in water in some areas. As a general rule, drink about 6 to 8 cups of water for hydration. Dietary sources of boron are excellent. However, one can overdose on supplemental boron. Boron could become toxic in high doses, use with care. Boron supplement may be available from your neighborhood drug store.

CALCIUM

Calcium is essential for the growth, maintenance and reproduction processes of the human body. Calcium is mainly known for its functions to maintain strong healthy bones and teeth of the body and for the prevention of the onset of osteoporosis. The attention catching property of calcium for consideration for this topic is the help it gives to the normal muscle contraction and relaxation cycle and its help in hormonal secretion. You can ingest Calcium as a supplement or from your daily diet. Plant sources include green leafy vegetables, kale and broccoli, beans and almonds. Animal sources of calcium include milk, yogurt and cheese. Calcium supplement is available over the counter from drug stores.

POTASSIUM

Potassium plays a role in metabolism and body functions such as acid-base regulation, muscle and body growth. It aids the muscle contraction and relaxation, and also very essential for proper blood circulation in the body system. Potassium helps the function of nitric oxide which also aids proper blood circulation in the innervation of blood vessels, blood capillaries and body cells and tissues.

It helps general circulation, innervation and blood supply to cells, tissues and muscle health.

Banana is particularly rich in potassium, manganese and magnesium. Other plant food sources rich in potassium include orange juice, vegetables such as sweet potatoes and Irish (including the back peel), squash, broccoli, and citrus fruits.

Animal sources of potassium include red meat, chicken, milk and seafood such as salmon, cod, and tuna.

PHOSPHOROUS

Phosphorous is required by nearly every cell and tissue of the body for optimal functioning. This is also very helpful, noting that deficiency in the body level of phosphorous may lead to muscle weakness, and anemia. Plant sources of phosphorous include almonds and peanuts. Animal food sources are milk, cheese, yogurt, eggs, and beef.

MANGANESE

Manganese is essential for the synthesis of fatty acids, which is necessary for a healthy nervous system. The nervous system is somewhat the electrical system of the body. The nervous system regulates the production and secretion of hormones.

ZINC

The Zinc is good for the production of testosterone, the sex hormone that boosts sexual desire, sexual arousal, sex drive and libido in both men and women. Zinc in combination with B vitamins is excellent for sperm count and fertility. Healthy zinc level in the body is same as healthy testosterone level in the body. Healthy testosterone level in the body (male and female) means high sex drive or high libido.

Zinc in combination with B6 and B9 (folate/folic acid) raises sperm production, motility, sperm count or semen volume and testosterone production. Low levels of zinc in the body system have been since linked to poor libido in men and women.

Zinc in combination with Vitamin B6 + Vitamin B9 + Selenium is very good for the good quality sperm production including sperm count/volume, sperm motility, sperm viability and virility.

COPPER

Copper has healing properties. Copper in conjunction with Vitamin C and Zinc provides an environment for the optimal production of elastin and elastin fibers. Increase intake of Zinc requires increased intake of copper. Copper is deeply involved in the electrical and transportation system of the body. It helps in the production of skin color or production of melanin, formation of red-blood cells, transportation and absorption of iron, transmission of electrical messages across neurons, formation of new blood vessels and blood capillaries, and helps to regulate blood pressure and heart beat. Copper in conjunction with zinc helps to prevent hair loss. Copper is a trace element and is needed in trace quantity by the body. Daily balanced diet may be able to supply daily body needs. Daily zinc intake also require copper intake to maintain a balance. When you take zinc, copper and vitamin c, you provide the most optimum environment for the skin production of elastin and collagen. Elastic and collagen are essential for the health and optimal functioning of vaginal muscle and penile fiber and muscle.

IRON

Iron is good for the formation of new blood cells. Adequate formation of blood cells aid circulation and nutrients are easily taken to destinations and in this case to the genitals. Red blood cells are good for transporting oxygen to the cells of the body including the tissues of the genitals. Adequate supply of oxygen is dependent on healthy blood platelets and in turn dependent on iron supply to the body blood system. An adequately aerated and fed genital cells and tissues is a healthy genital.

169

GENERAL BRIEF

It is a well-known fact albeit unspoken fact that the only logic in the bedroom is healthy and vibrant sex drive, sexual desire, sexual arousal and libido. In the general politics of any relationship, and marriage, the politics of the bedroom is the most vital. Guess Why? Because once you and your sex partner are happy each time you embark on your journey to heaven, to paradise, the rest of the drag that is existential in any relationship becomes manageable. All the points, methods, techniques, foods, vitamins and minerals outlined in this book are not quick fix. Maintaining a healthy and mindful lifestyle and incorporating the foods, herbs and exercise discussed in this edition of the book, in your daily way of life should be a primary focus. The understanding that it is a continuous course of duty and lifestyle will make the intake of these food, herbs, vitamins and minerals to be effective in increasing and maintaining your sexual health. For best result, articulate daily feeding with doing supplement and vitamins. Some of the herbs are better used on intermittent rather than on a daily basis. Again, as said earlier, the methods and techniques are not quick fix. However, some foods, herbs, vitamins and juices are better taken hours and minutes before any bedroom session. They take days, weeks, months and years to show a lasting effect. Good thing about the manifestation of the result/effect of the exercise and dietary regimen is that once they manifest, most people can hold on for as long as life permits. Why? Because the more you practice it, the more you will get used to maintaining the dietary lifestyle and regimen.

GLOSSARY OF TERMS

Anorgasmia – sexual arousal disorder that involves taking unusually long time or unable to achieve orgasm

Asexuality - lack of sexual attraction towards other people irrespective of gender

Sexual desire disorder – a disease or ailment that prevents an individual from having sexual desire

Sexual arousal disorder – a disease or ailment that prevents an individual from having sexual arousal including orgasm

Vaginal muscles – the muscles (flesh) lining the vaginal canal

Stratified – having layers, not a solid whole

Epithelial – membranous tissues of one or more layers of cells, always having protective or covering functions.

Nervi Erigentis – The nerve responsible for penile erection

Anterior wall – front wall

Posterior wall – back wall

Vaginal canal – the hole inside the vagina

Sub-mucosa – under the mucosa

Elastin – structural protein

Frigidity – a type of sexual arousal dysfunction, you may say a woman's version of erectile dysfunction

Vaginal muscularis – vaginal smooth muscles

PC muscle – Pelvic muscle (aka Love muscle)

Estrogen – female sex hormone (also present in men in smaller quantity)

Incontinence - inability to stop urine leakage from the bladder, the loss of control over the muscle that controls the bladder opening and closure

Latent Homosexuality – Unexpressed and never/suppressed homosexuality in an individual

Menopause – the phase when a woman stops seeing her menstrual cycle, stop ovulating.

Vaginal atrophy – the thinning and wasting away of the vaginal wall

Vasodilation - dilation or increase in the diameter of blood vessels

Vasoconstriction–Constriction or reduction in the size of the diameter of blood vessels

Structural changes – changes in the structure, shape, form

Bladder – the human urine sac

Bladder muscle – the muscle that controls the opening and closing of the bladder for the passage of urine

Rectal wall muscles – the muscles lining the rectal canal

Rectum – the tube through which stool is pushed out to the outside as you defecate

Vaginal Prolapse – vaginal collapse, when all the muscles became loose, and the bladder or rectum falls into the vaginal canal

Flatulence – outing of air

Vaginal Flatulence – expelling air from the vagina (vaginal farting)

Pleasure tunnel – vaginal canal

Pleasure canal – vaginal canal

Kegels – name given to vaginal wall muscle exercise as an attribute to Dr. Kegel who developed/discovered the exercise in the 1940's

Kegel Exercise - name given to vaginal wall muscle and PC muscle exercise as an attribute to Dr. Kegel who developed/discovered the exercise in the 1940's

Kegel balls – Devices and objects developed over the years to help target the exact PC muscle as you perform Kegels

Pelvic Floor - The pelvic floor is that point in the pelvic region of the body where all the connective tissues and muscles that support all the organs of the pelvis connects

Hormones – Bio-chemicals (chemicals of the body) in the body system that affects body changes and functions

Hormonal changes – changes in the levels of the body hormones

Sexual addiction - uncontrollable sexual outbursts, sexual behaviors and sexual thoughts

Testosterone – the male sex hormone, it helps give the male characteristics

Stinging Wasp – an insect

Symptom – manifested sign

Phytoestrogen – estrogens that are naturally present in plants

Estrogen-like chemicals – chemicals that resemble estrogen

Estrogenic activities – activities native to estrogens

Neurotransmitters – Body electrical transmitters

Omega-3 fatty acids – they are not acids in the common sense of the word acid. It is the name given to some essential fats that is good for the body system

Polyunsaturated Amino acids- long/multiple chain unsaturated amino acids

Monounsaturated amino acid – one chain unsaturated amino acid

Optimum hormonal level – perfect level for the body estrogen, a level at which it is at its best

Hormonal imbalance – imbalance of the levels of the hormones in the body system

Progesterone – a sex hormone present in both male and female body system, always more in males than females

Muscular contraction and relaxation – the ease and squeeze actions/movements of the body muscles

Roe – Fish eggs harvested for food (often unfertilized)

Sperm Count – The quantity and quality of sperm (semen volume)

Sperm Motility – The agility or mobility of sperm, ability to move towards the Ova to fertilize it.

ABOUT BE-YOUR-DREAM PRESS

BeYourDream Press is an imprint of Obrake USA LLC. We are publishers of non-fiction books. Books published by Be Your Dream Press are mainly books that help people to be whatever they want to be. Books that help people succeed in doing whatever legitimate thing they want to engage in.Be Your Dream Press publishes series of health and beauty books, women's health books and the very popular series called Financial Democracy Series.

Other Books by **BeYourDream Books** Include:

➢ Bedroom Justice

➢ Bedroom Fool

➢ Bedroom Wisdom

➢ Secrets To Skin Glow and Radiance

➢ Secrets To Hair Growth and Sheen

FINANCIAL DEMOCRACY SERIES

❖ A Manufacturer without A Factory

❖ Steps to Sell, Supply and Do Business with New York City

❖ Steps to Sell, Supply and Do Business with Large Corporations in America

❖ Steps to Sell, Supply and Do Business with Educational Institutions in America

❖ Steps to Sell, Supply and Do Business with International Institutions and Organizations

❖ Dozen Businesses You Can Start and Run in America

For more information visit us at: www.obrake.com/books

OTHER BOOKS BY **Be Your Dream Press**

FINANCIAL DEMOCRACY SERIES – CANADA
- ➢ Two Dozen Businesses You Can Start and Run in Canada
- ➢ No Canadian Experience

FINANCIAL DEMOCRACY SERIES – SOUTH AFRICA
- ❖ How to Sell, Supply and Do Business with National, Provincial, Local and Municipal Government of South Africa
- ❖ How to Sell, Supply and Do Business with Public and Private Corporations in South Africa
- ❖ How to Start and Run Your Business in South Africa
- ❖ Two Dozen Businesses You Can Start and Run in South Africa
- ❖ When South African Banks Say No

Visit us at: www.obrake.com/books

Bedroom Politics Series

BEDROOM LOGIC

Bedroom Logic = Sex Drive+ Sexual Desire+ Sexual Arousal +Libido

In the complex politics of a relationship, Bedroom Politics has a special hard-to-ignore and strategic position. In the politics of the bedroom, the only logical rally is healthy and vibrant sex drive, sexual desire, sexual arousal and libido.

It is therefore very important that you don't falter in this very important aspect of the politics of the bedroom. A low-libido partner, a low sex drive partner is an illogical partner and a Bedroom Fool.

Guess Why? Because once you and your sex partner are happy each time you embark on your journey to heaven, to paradise, the rest of the drag that is existential in any and all relationships becomes manageable.

Low Libido, weak sex drive, unhealthy sexual desire and sexual arousal may be caused by a variety of reasons. However, most causes of low libido and sex drive are manageable, reversible and curable.

Most of the cure and therapy exist in the Vitamins, Supplements, Foods and Fruits you see every day in your neighborhood grocery store. You only need to know them and how to combine them to assist you with your desire for a healthy sex drive and libido.

In this edition of the book, you will find:

➤ Foods to Improve Your Sex Drive
➤ Fruits to Enhance Your Libido
➤ Vitamins to Optimize You Sexual Desire
➤ Minerals to Heighten Your Sexual Arousal
➤ Supplements to Sustain Your Stamina
➤ All You Need to Intensify Your Orgasm

BE YOUR DREAM PRESS
www.obrake.com

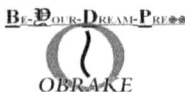

Be-Your-Dream-Press
OBRAKE

www.ingramcontent.com/pod-product-compliance
Lightning Source LLC
Chambersburg PA
CBHW020002290326
41935CB00007B/267